MEDICINE
BETRAYED

★

B M A

BRITISH MEDICAL ASSOCIATION

MEDICINE BETRAYED

THE PARTICIPATION OF DOCTORS IN
HUMAN RIGHTS ABUSES

★

Report of a Working Party

ZED BOOKS

in association with the

BMA

Medicine Betrayed was first published by Zed Books Ltd,
57 Caledonian Road, London N1 9BU, UK, and 165 First Avenue,
Atlantic Highlands, New Jersey 07716, USA, in association with
the British Medical Association, BMA House, Tavistock Square,
London WC1H 9JP, in 1992.

Cover designed by Andrew Corbett.
Typeset by Jaime Gales.
Printed and bound in the United Kingdom
by Biddles Ltd, Guildford and King's Lynn.

A catalogue record for this book is
available from the British Library

ISBN 1 85649 103 X Hb
ISBN 1 85649 104 8 Pb

This report is dedicated to the memory of Dr John Dawson (1946-1990) whose commitment to the defence of human rights and medical ethics was crucial to the role of the British Medical Association's activities in this field and to the effective functioning of the working parties which gave rise to the 1986 *Torture Report* and to this present report.

Acknowledgements

Individuals

We wish to thank the following for the assistance they gave in the Working Party's discussions and in the preparation of this report: Mrs Helen Bamber, Dr Adriaan van Es, Dr Blandine Geny, Dr Semyon Gluzman, Prof. Robert J Lifton, Dr Gregorio Martirena, Dr Mahboob Mehdi, Prof. Derrick Pounder, Dr Anne-Marie Raat, Prof. Michael Radelet, Nigel Rodley, Dr Gunter Seelman, Dr Peter Vesti plus others who gave us evidence on condition of anonymity.

In addition we want to acknowledge the courage shown by the many individuals whose testimony given to courts, inquiries, newspapers and journals, and human rights bodies has provided us with powerful evidence of the abuses we have discussed during the course of the Working Party enquiry.

Associations

The following associations responded to invitations from the BMA to submit evidence or comment: The Australian Medical Association, Colegio Médico de Chile, Danish Medical Association, Finnish Medical Association, Hong Kong Medical Association, Indian Medical Association, New Zealand Medical Association, Medical Association of South Africa, National Medical and Dental Association (South Africa), Royal Colleges of Nurses, Surgeons (London and Edinburgh), General Practitioners, and Physicians (United Kingdom), and the Colegio Médico Cubano Libre (USA).

In addition, the World Medical Association and the International Council of Nurses sent written information. We received much useful information from Amnesty International, Physicians for Human Rights, Johannes Wier Foundation, the Medical Foundation for the Care of Victims of Torture and many other organizations whose publications have contributed to this report.

Working Party Consultant: James Welsh

BMA Secretariat

Dr John Dawson (dec.)	Deborah Pippard
Dr Fleur Fisher	Ann Sommerville
Dr Natalie-Jane Macdonald	

Contents

	Dedication	v
	Acknowledgements	vi
	Foreword by Lord Avebury	x
	Preface	xiv
1	Introduction	1
2	Ethical standards and international law	9
	BMA policy	10
	International ethical standards	12
	International humanitarian law	15
	International human rights instruments/law	16
3	Assessing the evidence	20
	Torture: the scale of the problem	21
	Medical involvement in torture	25
	Abuse of psychiatry	30
	Corporal and capital punishments	31
	Conclusion	32
4	Medical involvement in torture	33
	Why do doctors get involved?	35
	How do doctors get involved?	40
	Assessing the evidence	42
	Examination prior to torture	42
	During torture	45
	After torture	49
	Pressure to assist in human rights violations	54
	Which doctors torture?	56
	Investigating medical involvement	59
	Conclusion	62
5	Abuse of psychiatry	64
	Evidence of psychiatric abuse	66
	Changes in Soviet law	68
	Visits of foreign experts, 1989-1991	69
	The rehabilitation process	72
	Other recent reports of psychiatric abuse	73
	Romania	73
	Cuba	74
	Germany	76
	Systematic failures in psychiatric practice	77
	Greece	77
	Japan	77
	United Kingdom	79
	Conclusion	80

6	Judicial penalties: corporal and capital punishment	83
	Corporal punishment	84
	National and international laws diverge	86
	Cultural values and medical involvement	93
	Cultural and religious values and corporal punishments	96
	Capital punishment	98
	Medical participation in capital punishment	102
	Contributing to the investigation phase	104
	Giving evidence in a capital trial	104
	Examining and certifying fitness	108
	Providing medical care to the prisoner	109
	Advising on, supervising or overseeing the punishment	111
	Certifying death	116
	Conclusions	117
7	Hunger strikes and other human rights issues involving prisoners	119
	Hunger strikes and forcible feeding	120
	The UK: evolution of policy	122
	Experiences outside the UK	125
	Forcible medication for non-medical reasons	131
	Withholding medical care	138
	Forcible examination of prisoners	141
	Forcible taking of blood or tissue samples	142
	Asylum seekers	143
	Other abuses in which doctors can participate	144
	Virginity testing	144
	Forcible sterilization	144
	Culturally-determined surgical procedures	145
	Experimentation on prisoners	146
	Trade in human organs	147
	Conclusion	148
8	Doctors as victims of repression	150
	How doctors come to be targeted	151
	Prosecution of opponents of psychiatric abuse: USSR	151
	Arrests in Syria	153
	Civil unrest: El Salvador	155
	Attack on human rights organization: Chile	157
	Arrest of health workers during mass demonstrations: China	158
	Criticism of government health policy: Vietnam	159
	Sudden change in government by coup: Sudan	160
	Humanitarian actions: Turkey	161
	Invasion: Kuwait	162
	Ethnic conflict: Yugoslavia	163
	Killings by opposition movements	164
	The need for international protection	165
9	The response of the medical profession	168
	Resistance to medical involvement	168

	Medical associations: the track record	168
	BMA activities	175
	The World Health Organization	176
	International Associations	177
	The role of other non-governmental organizations	180
	Proposal for an international tribunal	181
	The impossible dilemma - hero or victim	182
10	Monitoring the threat	184
	Declared respect for international standards	184
	The judiciary	186
	Police stations	187
	Prison practice	187
	Medical practice in prisons	189
	Mental health facilities	190
	Conclusion	190
11	Conclusions and recommendations	191
	Recommendations	194
	Involvement of doctors in torture	194
	Provision of medical care to prisoners and torture victims	196
	Treatment of hunger strikers	197
	Doctors working in the armed forces	197
	Support for doctors entering the prison service and armed forces	198
	Strengthening medical ethics	198
	Action by national medical associations	199
	Doctors and the death penalty	200
	Whipping and amputations	201
	The role of forensic medicine	203
	Protection of health professionals	203
	Care for victims of human rights violations	204
	Other issues	205
	Further action	206
Appendices		207
1.	BMA activities on human rights issues	207
2.	Resolutions passed at BMA Annual Representative Meetings	208
3.	WMA: Declaration of Tokyo	210
4.	WMA: Resolution on physician participation in capital punishment	211
5.	WMA: Declaration in hunger-strikers	212
6.	WPA: Declaration of Hawaii	215
7.	WPA: Declaration on psychiatrists and the death penalty	217
8.	UN Principles of Medical Ethics	217
9.	12 point program of Amnesty International	220
10.	UK ratification of international conventions	221
Bibliography		223
Index		228

Foreword

The most remarkable, and counter-intuitive, fact about torture is that it is practised mainly by apparently ordinary men, and a few ordinary women as well. Milgram showed that it was possible to set up conditions in which ordinary Americans could be persuaded to torture fellow human beings[1], and the evidence shows that in the main, the torturers of Argentina in the 1970s, and Sudan or Sri Lanka in the present day, were not psychopaths but family men who considered they were doing their patriotic duty in a life and death combat against dangerous enemies of society.

Doctors, because of their training in the prevention of suffering, and their commitment to a code of ethics involving the preservation of human life, might be expected to show a much greater resistance than others to the pressures which cause people to harm others deliberately, and in democratic states with a traditional respect for human rights, there is little evidence of direct involvement of doctors in torture or ill-treatment of detainees. The problems that do arise are those of forcible medication, force feeding and lack of care, rather than deliberate ill-treatment.

In the UK, there has been public concern about deaths in custody, ranging from the case of Barry Prosser[2] who was unlawfully killed in Winson Green prison at one extreme, to the spate of suicides in Brixton. In some of these cases there has been evidence of a lack of care. From time to time there are also allegations of the use of medication[3] as an instrument of control, and the huge differences in prescribing patterns of psychotropic drugs among prisons cannot be accounted for by clinical factors. The facilities for treatment of seriously mentally ill patients in prisons are grossly inadequate. Reception medical facilities are often

---

1 Milgram S. Behavioral study of obedience. *Journal of Abnormal Social Psychology*, 1963; **67**:277-85.

2 Coroner to send inquest report to DPP after jury decides that prisoner was unlawfully killed, *The Times*, 14 April 1981.

3 Freeman v Home Office. *Weekly Law Reports*, 1979 F No 1449, 11 May 1984.

filthy and lacking in privacy, and the Prison Medical Directorate's statistics on HIV, drug abuse, hypertensives and diabetics are likely to be unreliable. As the Chief Inspector of Prisons has said, "the standard of medical care afforded to prisoners falls far short of that provided in the community" and "can only diminish further"[4].

All the same, there is, of course, a huge difference between the neglect and complacency of the Prison Department here in Britain, and the deliberate infliction of harm on detainees which is seen under some regimes, and not only dictatorships. In Sri Lanka, El Salvador, Guatemala, India and Turkey, for instance, elections are held regularly and yet there are persistent reports of torture and ill-treatment. From 1983 to 1991, the UN Human Rights Commission recorded as many as 12,000 persons having disappeared in Sri Lanka[5], many of them after being detained in police stations or camps. Under the Emergency Regulations, the authorities could dispose of dead bodies without any formal proceedings, but if any of the thousands of murders by the police and security forces did come to the notice of Judicial Medical Officers (JMO), whose duties included those of coroner, they were not reported except in the very rare cases where there were court proceedings. In one notorious case, where a human rights lawyer had been severely tortured in the Assistant Superintendent of Police's private house in Matara, the victim was brought back to the capital, Colombo, in response to a writ of habeas corpus, but he died in the Colombo General Hospital the same evening, before he could be produced in court. The JMO who gave evidence at the inquest understated the extent of the deceased's injuries, but corrected himself under cross examination[6].

The Declaration of Tokyo implicitly requires a doctor to denounce any cases of torture which come to his or her notice, something of a counsel of perfection. Some of the lawyers who took up human rights cases in Sri Lanka were themselves murdered, and many others had to flee the country in fear of their lives. In Sudan, doctors who protested against the repression by the "Revolutionary Command Council" in November 1989 were arrested on charges of high treason, which carried

---

4 *Report of Her Majesty's Chief Inspector of Prisons - January 1990 - March 1991*. London: HMSO. ISBN 0-10-205492-4.

5 UN Commission on Human Rights. Report of the Working Group on Enforced or Involuntary Disappearances. Addendum. Doc. E/CN.4/1992/18/Add.1, 8 January 1992, para.185. The Group noted that the cases recorded for Sri Lanka represent "by far the highest number ever recorded by the Working Group for any single country" [para.192].

6 High Court Case No 3715/88, Colombo, Sri Lanka.

the death penalty. In Chile, Dr Sheila Cassidy, a British doctor who had merely treated victims of torture, was herself arrested and tortured[7] - one of a number who suffered such a fate. There are probably hundreds of doctors living in Britain as exiles, because they were persecuted for opposing torture and other human rights abuses in their countries of origin[8], and unfortunately more are still arriving.

In states or territories which are effectively cut off from the rest of the world, such as Burma or Tibet, opposition by doctors to torture or ill-treatment would be even more quixotic.

When doctors are wholly or mainly drawn from the dominant ethnic or national group, and the victims are from a minority, there may be special dangers. In Tibet, detainees who reported on the practice of compulsory blood extraction mentioned that Chinese doctors were responsible. In East Timor, all the doctors come from outside the occupied territory. An East Timorese who gave evidence to the UN Sub-Commission on Prevention of Discrimination and Protection of Minorities in August 1991, Paulino Game, said that he was interrogated by Indonesian doctors, who used electric shock torture, and he gave the name of the head of the medical team involved, who claimed to have been trained in the United States. In the Yugoslavian province of Kosovo, almost all doctors and other health professionals of Albanian ethnic origin were dismissed after July 1990, and partially replaced by young, inexperienced personnel from Serbia[9]. In Kashmir, it has been reported that Indian army doctors removed a kidney from a young Kashmiri detainee[10].

As in all other human rights problems, so it is with the participation of doctors in torture and other inhuman treatment of detainees: much useful work has been done on standards, but far too little on enforcement. Until recently, the doctrine of non-intervention in the internal affairs of member states, enshrined in the UN Charter, has severely limited the scope for action either by Governments or NGOs on serious violations of accepted norms, including the UN's Convention Against Torture and other Cruel, Inhuman or Degrading Treatment of

---

7   *Guardian*, 20 February 1975.

8   *BMA New Review*, 4(1); January 1978.

9   Dr Werner Vogt, Prof. Erik Siesby & David Abraham. *The Health Care Situation in Kosovo*. International Helsinki Federation for Human Rights, Vienna, October 1991.

10 Ghulam Nabi Khayal. Boy says Soldiers removed his Kidney. Kashmir Council for Human Rights, 19 January 1992.

1984. States may refuse admission to persons seeking to investigate allegations of torture and, even where authoritative reports are published by newspapers or NGOs, the transgressor state suffers no material penalty.

Recently, however, there has been a growing debate on "The Right to Intervene", which may be defined as the right to deliver international humanitarian assistance across borders without the consent of the target state. Mme Georgina Dufoix, for example, writes of the principle as being "in keeping with a political will which aims to prevent or stop situations which are intolerable from a humanitarian point of view", and she cites Security Council Resolution 688 on the Kurds of northern Iraq as an example[11]. The G7 Declaration issued by the London Summit in July 1991 urged the UN and its agencies to be ready to consider similar action in the future if the circumstances require it and, whilst a military operation on the scale of the Gulf War might be an inappropriate response to gross and persistent use of torture in a state, the willingness of the United Nations to intervene in major world crises ought to be paralleled by a corresponding increase in the level of activity by private organisations to combat human rights violations.

This study, building on the previous work of the BMA on torture, comes to grips with the ethical and practical issues involved, and concludes with a set of specific recommendations. Among the most important of these is the establishment of an international procedure for reviewing cases where doctors are pressured into collusion with torture or maltreatment, and for developing international sanctions against the authorities responsible. Such an initiative would be fully in keeping with the deployment of a governmental "right to intervene", and would be a lasting memorial to the life and work of John Dawson.

Lord Avebury
Chairman
Parliamentary Human Rights Group

---

11 Mme Georgina Dufoix. The Right to Intervene. *Red Cross Red Crescent*, September-December 1991.

Preface

> What do you mean people don't care about torture? We'll make them care.[1]

That this report and its predecessor came to be written by a medical association owes much to the energies of Dr John Dawson. He headed the British Medical Association's International Division until his death in 1990 and was a linchpin in the development of the Association's human rights policy. This is not to underestimate, however, the considerable work undertaken by the members of two BMA Working Parties who have sifted the evidence, nor the powerful impetus from the BMA membership to pursue such work. Ultimately, it is the interests of members which keep subjects like human rights abuses constantly on the Association's agenda, and the extent of their interest is evidenced by the resolutions passed year upon year at the Association's annual meetings (ARMs).

Urgency has been given to the evolution of BMA policy by intermittent but persistent reports of the involvement of doctors in procedures which breach accepted standards for the treatment of detainees. In response, the BMA has adopted a wide range of policy decisions applicable to medical involvement in human rights abuses and related issues: since the early 1970s the Association has publicly condemned the abuse of medical or psychiatric skills. At the annual meetings in 1984 and 1986, resolutions were passed pledging BMA support to medical associations and to individual doctors who need help to resist such involvement. In 1991 several resolutions on prison issues were adopted. A list of some of the the relevant resolutions is appended to this report.

The 1984 meeting also recommended that the BMA Council should:

> set up a working party to investigate claims that, in some countries, doctors are co-operating with the use of torture as a routine instrument of repression by governments of all political persuasion.

---

1 John Dawson. From a profile published in *Physicians for Social Responsibility Quarterly*, 1991; **1**(3).

This gave rise to the first BMA report on the involvement of doctors in torture, which was published in 1986. The report concluded that there was "incontrovertible evidence of doctors' involvement in planning and assisting in torture, not only under duress, but also voluntarily as an exercise of the doctor's free will". It found not only varying degrees of involvement in maltreatment of prisoners but also collusion in the wrongful detention of healthy individuals in psychiatric facilities. It made a number of recommendations for positive steps to limit or prevent such activity in the future.

One of the practical elements of the report's conclusions was that there should be consistent, international, standards of ethics. In addition, the report concluded that it is wrong to give anybody medical skills and knowledge without, at the same time, putting these skills and knowledge into a framework of ethics that will constrain the way in which they are used. The final conclusions centred on the need to distance physicians from the state: the need to ensure that the physician's skills are not used in such a way that the medical profession becomes an agent of the state.

The Association was not under any illusion, however, that the problem of medical involvement in torture had been addressed or even recognised in its entirety. Moreover, the ethical problems posed by other forms of ill-treatment, and various punishments which continue to be applied, needed addressing. Thus, at the 1989 annual meeting, a further resolution was passed:

> That this Meeting views with great concern continuing reports of the abuses of medical skills in relation to prisoners, and asks Council to establish a working party to follow up the torture report, to examine new evidence, and to make appropriate recommendations.

This resulted, in 1990, in the establishment of the present Working Party, which comprised:

Sir Douglas Black: Past President, British Medical Association (Chairman);

Dr James Birley, CBE: Chairman, Special Committee on Unethical Practices in Psychiatry (SCOUPP); then President, Royal College of Psychiatrists;

Dr JS Horner: Chairman, BMA Medical Ethics Committee; Director of Public Health, Preston;

Prof I Kennedy: Barrister; Head and Dean of School of Law, Director of Centre of Medical Law and Ethics, Professor of Medical Law and Ethics, Kings College, London;

Prof B Knight: Barrister; Professor of Forensic Pathology, University of Wales College of Medicine, Cardiff;

Dr AW Macara: Chairman, BMA Representative Body; Consultant Senior Lecturer, Department of Epidemiology and Public Health Medicine, University of Bristol;

Dr Hernán Reyes: Medical Division, International Committee of the Red Cross, Geneva;

Dr Anne Rodway: Vice-chairman, BMA Medical Ethics Committee; General Practitioner;

Dr Michael Thomas: BMA Board of Science.

Guided by the ARM resolution, the Working Party adopted the following terms of reference for its study:

> To consider the circumstances under which torture and medical involvement in it occurs. To examine the role of doctors in torture, judicial and extra-judicial punishments. To examine the involvement of doctors in abuses of human rights[2]. To consider what health professionals can do to prevent the continued abuse of human rights and to alleviate the suffering of abused people. To make recommendations for action.

After careful consideration, the Working Party adopted the definition of torture which had been used for the 1984 report:

> Torture is the deliberate, systematic or wanton infliction of physical and mental suffering by one or more persons acting alone or on the orders of an authority, to force another person to yield information, to make a confession, or for any other reason which is an outrage on personal dignity.[3]

Over a two-year period, from January 1990 to late 1991, the Working Party received a wide range of written and oral testimony, some of which has been included in the report. In addition, interviews with individual doctors and representatives of national medical associations were carried out abroad on behalf of the Working Party and extensive research into the published literature was undertaken. It has not been

---

2   These were modified slightly during the work of the Working Party: investigations of human rights violations and extrajudicial punishments were restricted to those applicable to prisoners.

3   British Medical Association. *Torture Report*. 1986, p.4.

possible to reflect every case and issue submitted to the group but attempts have been made to give a representative selection and to include specific examples, where appropriate, throughout the report.

Full details of the method of evidence collection and verification are included in chapters 1 and 3. As with the previous BMA investigation, missions were not undertaken by the Working Party members specifically for this report. Assessment of the validity of evidence was helped considerably by the contributions of reputable human rights monitoring bodies and medical groups working for torture victims. The experiences of Amnesty International, the British and US branches of Physicians for Human Rights, the Johannes Wier Foundation, Netherlands and the American Association for the Advancement of Science, all of which have conducted many fact-finding missions by forensic and other experts, have helped the Working Party particularly with respect to assessing the reliability of information provided. The Medical Foundation for the Care of Victims of Torture in London, which receives detailed testimony from torture victims in the course of its work, contributed much evidence of its own experiences. The Working Party thanks all these groups for their help in the preparation of this report.

Finally, the Working Party wishes to express its admiration for those doctors and other health professionals who have striven to maintain their professional integrity despite living in circumstances where human rights violations are a daily reality. The members thank them for giving the benefit of their experiences and insights.

Chapter 1

Introduction

... he took my arm and very smoothly [said]: "You know Jacobo that we doctors have many secrets ... You see here: this blue is one of your arteries and I can inject here. You know that we have some substances that make you talk but it is always so painful because it affects your brain; so why can't you just talk and we can be friends".

His presence was terrible because he was the symbol that a scientific instrument is with you when you are tortured by the beasts.

(Jacobo Timerman, Argentinian writer)[1]

The practice of medicine confers both privileges and obligations. Medical skills are taught with the highest ideals in mind but unless mastery of the techniques is accompanied by knowledge and observance of the ethical obligations, those skills may be subverted as the testimony of Jacobo Timerman dramatically illustrates. Individuals who are held by the state are in a powerless and vulnerable position. Governments therefore have particular obligations to guarantee the safety and health of those they hold. Doctors, of course, play an important role in affirming those guarantees. The medical profession must be gravely concerned by reports of medical involvement in the deliberate maltreatment of detainees.

It is important to note that, contrary to the popular image, torture is not solely a repressive technique directed against political activists, whether violent or peaceful[2]. One of the many arguments made against torture is precisely that the target population — "enemies of the state" for example — has a way of growing. A manifesto of an Argentinean death squad illustrates this inflationary effect of extra-legal measures in a chilling manner: apart from desiring the "extermination" of communist cells and revolutionary groups it also sought to wipe out

---

1 Interview in *Doctors and Torture*. BBC television. (Producer: H Nazareth; Director: G Lanning) 12 September 1990.

2 Countries such as Mexico, Brazil, Turkey, India and many others are reported to use torture as an adjunct to criminal investigation. Details can be found in the annual *Amnesty International Reports*.

"common killers, robbers, assailants, rapists, homosexuals, prostitutes, drug addicts, military traitors, corrupt lawyers..."[3]. In some countries torture is used systematically to gain convictions in criminal cases, sometimes after the use of torture has been institutionalised during periods of political repression.

In chapter 2 we set out the national and international legal and ethical framework governing the work of doctors. There is a surprisingly extensive array of conventions, treaties, principles, declarations and codes which are relevant to the doctor. While we are under no illusion that statements of principle are a simple answer to major human rights problems we believe that, provided they are monitored, they do place constraints on those wishing to abuse prisoners and provide a useful basis on which to assess the behaviour of individuals, associations and states.

Any discussion of torture must be firmly based on the evidence available. Although it is persistently reported by international bodies and specialised monitoring groups, governments are not generally willing to admit to its use. The UN Special Rapporteur on Torture has also drawn attention to the fact that few governments will attempt to argue that torture is acceptable, more generally denying its existence or trying to find excuses to minimize its significance[4]. Some regimes, however, are probably not unhappy that information about torture circulates at home as it works as an intimidatory measure fostering rumour and uncertainty, as it is intended to do.

By its nature, torture undermines the individual's sense of security and self-worth. Victims may experience feelings of shame, guilt and self-doubt. It is certain that the incidence of torture is under-reported. Even when verified by physical examination, individual testimony is sometimes only available in generalised terms, as victims seek to protect themselves from the anguish of their experience or to protect others who might be put at risk by full disclosure of evidence. All of these factors pose obstacles to informed discussion of the subject. The inherent difficulties in obtaining and weighing the evidence in a responsible manner are explored in chapter 3 of this report.

---

3   Cited in: Guest I. *Behind the Disappearances: Argentina's Dirty War against Human Rights and the United Nations*. Philadelphia: University of Pennsylvania Press, 1990, note 7, p.511.

4   Professor Peter Kooijmans, UN Special Rapporteur on Torture; address at conference on "Torturers and their Masters", organised by the Project for the Inter-Disciplinary Study of Human Rights Violations (PIOOM), Leiden, Netherlands, 11 October 1991.

In the following chapter we examine how medical personnel are involved in torture. Doctors may be called upon to examine prisoners prior to torture to estimate fitness to withstand torture or identify weak points to be exploited. They may monitor the torture process to provide resuscitation or advice when a life-threatening limit is reached. Finally they may provide medical treatment after torture. This may either be part of ethical prison medical care, or may be to allow the prisoner to be publicly seen or to permit further maltreatment at a later date. Clearly, the latter practice is unethical.

Less direct involvement can occur when doctors issue inaccurate or deliberately falsified death certificates, perhaps without having requested, or been allowed, sight of the body. When a prisoner is released, inaccurate or deliberately falsified certification of fitness may be produced, again possibly without the prisoner having been medically examined. Again, we believe that such actions are contrary to medical ethics.

In chapter 4 we also consider what motivates doctors to become involved in abuses. In some cases they are subject to overt pressure: they may be called on to undertake obligatory military service and disobedience to a military command may risk serious consequences. A Chilean colleague explained to us the kind of pressures or physical threats which may be used and the desperate sense of isolation experienced by doctors who wish to refuse to submit to those pressures operating in a closed society. Other factors lead to medical complicity in torture. These include ideological sympathies with the objectives of the torturers. In some cases exaggerated accounts of the danger of particular prisoners, combined with the social marginalisation of particular social or political groups, can lead to individuals being regarded as "sub-human" and subsequently stripped of all rights. Testimony has also been given about the gradual and confused slide into participation by doctors who begin by attempting to help prisoners and only later become aware of the extent to which they have become compromised. At the end of the report, we have attempted to define measures which would deal with some of these problems.

Undeniably, there has been a great deal of international political change since the BMA published its previous report and some element of this is seen in the differing evidence available to the BMA torture working parties in the mid-1980s and in 1990-91. Military and other regimes without public accountability provide the circumstances which allow abuses to arise. Allegations of medical involvement in torture received by the previous working party primarily concerned such regimes in Latin America. Now Argentina, Chile and Uruguay have civilian governments. The focus has shifted to military and repressive governments in other regions, though abuses continue to occur in democratic states, as will be noted in chapter 4. During the period of our discussions, enormous changes have taken place in Eastern Europe particularly. While it is impossible yet to evaluate the tragic events of the war in Yugoslavia, for example, or the truth of allegations made against doctors caught up in the conflict, it is clear that widespread atrocities have occurred, some on hospital premises. Changes have also occurred in relation to the incarceration of healthy individuals in psychiatric facilities for political, religious or ethnic reasons. Such abuse has been documented in some countries with systematic political control of psychiatric medicine. It is alleged to have occurred in Czechoslovakia, Hungary, Romania and Yugoslavia and, according to recent reports, East Germany and Cuba, but has been best documented in the former USSR.

In the 1980s, political developments in the Soviet Union led to legislative change in the supervision of psychiatric hospitals and to potentially greater protection for the individual. During the time that the Working Party considered these matters, many questioned whether such hesitant progress could be developed in the face of decades of only minor change in the Soviet ideology of psychiatric practice and little change of personnel. In the latter months of our deliberations, profound political change has overtaken the Soviet Union and the results of this remain to be seen. The Ukrainian psychiatrist, Semyon Gluzman, who addressed the Working Party in person in 1990 and later through correspondence, strongly believed that the failure of Soviet officials to acknowledge the past extent of the political abuse of psychiatry had serious implications for the future. In October 1991, however, it appeared that the situation might be changing. The psychiatric internment and "treatment" of one noted dissident, General Piotr Grigorenko, was publicly acknowledged to have been unjustified by the Soviet authorities. It might have been thought that Grigorenko's posthumous rehabilitation might be the precursor of a systematic programme of rehabilitation of former victims of the abuses of past decades. However, progress is extremely slow and the political turmoil of the latter phase of the Gorbachev era and the establishment of the new Commonwealth are certain to slow things down in the immediate period.

In addition to the gross violations represented by torture and abuse of psychiatry for political reasons, we have considered punishments specified by law which involve doctors. Both corporal and capital punishments pose major ethical questions for the medical profession since they risk making doctors the arbiters of painful, or lethal, punishments. We have tried to evaluate in chapter 6 the extent to which doctors can be regarded as behaving unethically in their involvement in the execution of such punishments.

There is a wide range of government measures applied in some countries to the general public or the prison population which might be considered abuses of human rights. Only a small number of these have featured prominently in our discussions. In chapter 7, forced feeding of prisoners on hunger strike, administration to detainees of medication without clinical indication and punitive measures with health implications for prisoners are among the subjects discussed.

The Working Party takes a very firm view that any infringement of the dignity of the individual is a matter for concern and may eventually indicate a potential for serious abuse. We are greatly in sympathy with remarks by the UN Special Rapporteur on Torture, Professor Peter Kooijmans, that the international prohibition on torture may not be the most fundamental of rights — that the prohibition of an entire spectrum of degrading practices which fall short of torture underpin the concept of inherent human dignity[5]. In our discussions, therefore, much effort has been given to considering how to address the compromises and indignities visited upon some groups of vulnerable patients in our own country. Regretfully, we have considered it beyond the scope of this Working Party to adequately evaluate medical involvement in such infringements of the human rights of the public at large. We have not sought or evaluated the evidence of allegations of forcible sterilisation programmes, state pressure to restrict population growth through, for example, forcing women to have abortions, or official prohibition of contraceptive materials to increase population. Nor have we considered medical participation in cultural practices such as female circumcision. Although such issues have significant implications for doctors and are of serious concern, they are qualitatively different to the largely secret and unacknowledged government maltreatment of detainees.

Furthermore, we acknowledge the problem but cannot address in any more than a superficial way in this report, the appalling conditions in some geriatric and psychiatric units, where little or no medical attention is given to residents. During the period of our discussions, punitive and "therapeutic" practices in residential children's homes in England and Wales have also come under severe criticism. We feel that there is a

---

5   Address by Professor Kooijmans at conference on "Torturers and their Masters", *op. cit.*

clear protective role for medical practitioners to fulfil in such institutions, but that this is for others to address in detail.

Balancing our profound concern about doctors' involvement in maltreatment of prisoners and administration of judicial punishments, is a very deep anxiety about doctors who themselves suffer torture and execution. It must be stressed that among this group there are some who are detained and tortured as a result of their attempts to stop human rights abuses and to help victims of torture. But it is not only those who are thought to be helping torture victims who in turn become victims themselves. In some countries, educated professionals such as doctors, lawyers and teachers are seen as, or may in fact be, opponents of the government and are amongst the first to attract persecution. In Sudan, for example, doctors and civil servants were detained after the military coup of 30 June 1989. Amongst those arrested in the course of that year were Dr Ali Fadul, who reportedly died under torture while detained by the military, and Dr Mohamed Hussain who was sentenced to death for his involvement in a ten minute discussion to plan a doctors' strike[6]. In Syria also, a large number of doctors and lawyers were arrested in 1980 after a strike organised in support of basic human rights and for an end to State of Emergency regulations. The strike was led by the Syrian Bar Association and was supported by the Medical Association and other professional groups. More than 90 health workers were held imprisoned without trial in poor conditions for more than a decade and may still be in detention; despite a large number of releases of prisoners promised in late 1991, no information on the fate of the imprisoned medical personnel has been released by the Syrian government.

Such cases pose major questions concerning the role of associations such as the BMA in supporting ethical actions by doctors under threat. In chapter 9 we have attempted to assess the extent to which medical associations have acted to defend human rights and medical ethics and to give protection to threatened health professionals.

Despite the difficulties, a wide range of written and oral testimony has been received by the Working Party and reference to specific cases has been included wherever relevant. Before undertaking this study, the Working Party sought information from all national medical associations, human rights organisations in many countries among the

---

6 Dr Hussain's death sentence was commuted and he was released in May 1990, immediately prior to the arrival in Khartoum of a two-member delegation representing US human rights and professional organizations.

best known of which is Amnesty International, and specialised medical human rights groups such as the various national branches of Physicians for Human Rights. The Medical Foundation for the Care of Victims of Torture kindly supplied copies of testimony gained through its work with torture victims. The experiences of other centres have also been taken account of where they have published relevant material.

We are also grateful to a number of organisations and individuals who responded to our invitation to present oral evidence. In addition to the previously mentioned organisations, oral evidence was presented by experts in Soviet abuse of psychiatry and psychiatric involvement in death penalty decisions in the USA. Doctors who witnessed part of the process which led to maltreatment of political prisoners in Chile and Uruguay have also recounted their experiences. Evidence on corporal punishment and torture in Pakistan was given by a colleague from that country.

Although this report concentrates on cases where doctors have been involved, the available evidence suggests that these are a minority of all reported torture incidents since much torture appears to take place without doctors present. The aims of this Working Party have not included attempts to form a definitive assessment of the scale of torture nor of medical involvement. We believe such assessments must largely be a matter for informed conjecture for reasons discussed in chapter 3. We have considered whether medical participation in maltreatment has changed since the BMA's previous report and have regretfully concluded that, while some of the places may have changed, the spectrum of abuses unfortunately remains the same. Our main purpose, however, has been to look at how and why doctors become involved and, more importantly, how this might be prevented.

In preparing this report, we have been dismayed by the evidence of the scale and magnitude of the ill-treatment deliberately inflicted. Even more disturbing is the degree of involvement of some doctors. While clearly recognising the immense pressures to which some have been subject, it is also clear to us that others have involved themselves in disreputable practices with little forethought.

What is profoundly difficult for the profession to accept is the apparently voluntary participation of doctors in some circumstances. Perhaps some brief remarks by a German doctor, recently giving a paper about human rights abuses in the former German Democratic Republic, summarise what we have found to be the most disturbing aspect of medical participation:

It is clear that they were not monsters who worked there. Most doctors were probably just doing their job as far as they could. Some were collaborators, others just informed the Stasi about the talks people had in their lunch-breaks. It didn't have to be a really dangerous thing.... They didn't have to do it. To say no, you didn't have to be a hero.[7]

In conclusion, the evidence of both the involuntary and the voluntary participation of doctors in a range of human rights violations must spur the profession to give urgent consideration to preventive measures. The recommendations at the end of this report reflect our deliberations on this matter.

---

7 Dr Claudia Malzfeldt. Victims of Stasi repression and how to deal with colleagues who worked for the Stasi. Paper given at an international symposium on "Health and Human Rights in Eastern Europe", Amsterdam, Johannes Wier Foundation, 1 November 1991.

Chapter 2

Ethical standards and international law

Is it not a pleasant tribute to the medical profession that by and large it has been able to manage its relations with its patients ... without the aid of lawyers and lawmakers?[1]

Notwithstanding the optimistic comments of Lord Devlin, an understanding of legal, ethical and human rights standards is essential to any analysis of doctors' relationships to prisoners and other vulnerable detained individuals. The function of this chapter is to establish the legal and ethical basis of the unacceptability of medical involvement in human rights abuses and to provide a framework for the report of the Working Party.

The behaviour of doctors is guided by laws and ethical codes of different levels of immediacy and force. The first and most immediate are the laws and ethical codes applying in the country in which the doctor practises. Some countries have a range of laws which regulate aspects of medical training, practice, research and working conditions. In addition, the medical profession itself — either through regulatory bodies or through voluntary professional bodies such as medical associations — sets out detailed codes of conduct intended to regulate most aspects of medical practice including those areas where the doctor may affect the rights of others. This is most sharply seen in the relationship between the doctor and the prisoner, since the latter has been, by virtue of the judicial process, stripped of the right of liberty and various other rights which are protected for the free citizen.

It is of note that there is no regime of legal principles in Britain which specifically regulates the doctor-patient relationship. Nor are there any provisions in the law of any part of the UK dealing specifically with the doctor's obligations to respect human rights beyond

---

1 Lord Devlin in his Lloyds Robert Lecture to the Medical Society of London (Samples of Lawmaking, 1962, *Medicine and the Law* 83:103).

those inherent in the regulatory framework of medical practice and those applicable to the general public. This is probably the case in other countries though in Argentina, for example, legislation was introduced in February 1984 which made the failure of an official to report torture punishable by a prison sentence of between one and five years. The law provided that "if the official is a doctor the period of imprisonment will be doubled and he will be barred from exercising his profession". This provision is now part of the Argentine Penal Code[2].

In the UK, the statutory body, the General Medical Council, does not give specific guidance on medical involvement in human rights abuses in its publication on professional conduct and discipline of the British medical profession[3]. It does, however, include much general advice on behaviour which might constitute serious professional misconduct and lead to the removal of the doctor's name from the medical register. Such behaviour includes disregard by doctors of their professional responsibilities to patients for their care and treatment, abuse of professional skills and conduct derogatory to the reputation of the medical profession.

BMA policy

The British Medical Association's clear policy is that medical ethics prohibit any involvement by doctors in torture and that doctors in countries where torture does not occur have a responsibility to assist colleagues in countries where it does. The Association has also adopted some specific guidance on some of the human rights issues under discussion in this report.

Torture and other cruel, inhuman or degrading treatment or punishment: In the BMA's publication *Philosophy and Practice of Medical Ethics* (1988), guidance is given on the doctor's ethical response to torture. Torture is seen to involve much more than the physical abuse of prisoners. It is an outrage on personal dignity. The BMA regards any such outrage as abhorrent and the involvement of doctors, directly or indirectly, as unethical.

---

2 Cited in Amnesty International. *Argentina: Doctor convicted of torture released under "due obedience" law.* AI Index: AMR 13/10/87, 17 December 1987.

3 General Medical Council. *Professional Conduct and Discipline: Fitness to Practice.* London: GMC, 1991.

The publication draws heavily on the findings and recommendations of the Association's *Torture Report* (1986). Not only does it make clear the absolute prohibition on medical involvement in torture, including the presence of a doctor during the interrogation of a prisoner, *Philosophy and Practice of Medical Ethics* also addresses the issue of medical *acquiescence* in torture or other abuses. It states:

> During the course of his duties a doctor may witness abuses.... He may not be directly involved but may by chance have seen some incident on his way to or from his patient. The doctor will first need to assess the nature and severity of the abuse. Having decided that the matter should be pursued, the doctor will then need to decide whether to make further enquiries and possibly to register a formal protest within the organisation, or whether the matter is so serious that his protest must be registered outside the institution. *It is unethical for the doctor to tolerate a situation which he knows to be wrong even if the discovery was entirely accidental.* [p.38; emphasis added.]

It sees the doctor's obligations as also embodying a *positive* obligation and reiterates recommendations of the earlier Torture Working Party, stating:

> Doctors having knowledge of any activities covered by the [World Medical Association's] *Declaration of Tokyo* have a positive obligation to make those activities publicly known. [p.37]

and:

> The medical profession has a responsibility to support any practitioner who refuses to keep silent about abuses of human rights.... Doctors in countries where torture does not occur have a responsibility to assist colleagues in countries where it does. [p.37]

With regard to use of medical drugs on detainees, the BMA has always stressed its view that it is unethical for a doctor to administer a drug to a prisoner for any purpose other than for his or her clinical care. In its chapter dealing with medical involvement in torture, *Philosophy and Practice of Medical Ethics* classifies as assisting in torture "the administration of drugs which have no therapeutic purpose and which may positively harm the subject" [p.36].

Judicial punishments: The BMA Handbooks of Medical Ethics published in the early and mid-1980s set out the ethical principles, which the Association still maintains, governing the doctor's role in the administration of punishment. With respect to restricted diet, the

Association states in these publications that "any diet so restricted that medical monitoring is necessary … is inhuman, and no doctor should be associated with it."[4] It notes that "a doctor would be acting unethically if he certified a prisoner as fit to undergo [corporal punishment or incarceration in a dark cell]. Attendance at the corporal punishment of a prisoner is unethical."[5]

Forcible feeding of hunger-strikers: The BMA debated the issue of the artificial feeding of prisoners in 1974. It concluded that the practice was distinctly different from torture for reasons which included the conscientiously-held beliefs of some within the profession to do all in their power to preserve life. The situation was clarified in the following year when the BMA was a prime mover of the World Medical Association's Declaration of Tokyo which included at paragraph 5 that prisoners capable of forming a rational judgement about the consequences of hunger strike should not be fed artificially without consent. The BMA maintains this position.

International ethical standards

At regional and international levels, professional bodies have adopted ethical guidelines intended to reflect regional or universal values and which embody an ethical consensus. They therefore have a powerful moral force if not legal enforceability. Of these standards, the most explicit standard proscribing medical involvement in torture is the World Medical Association's *Declaration of Tokyo*. Adopted in 1975, it states, in its first paragraph, that:

> the doctor shall not countenance, condone or participate in the practice of torture or other forms of cruel, inhuman or degrading procedures, whatever the offence of which the victim of such procedures is suspected, accused or guilty, and whatever the victim's beliefs or motives, and in all situations, including armed conflict and civil strife.

It goes on to define further the forms of involvement prohibited under the Declaration (such as providing premises or knowledge), to prohibit attendance at torture, to insist on complete clinical independence *vis-à-vis* the patient, to prohibit forcible feeding where the prisoner can make a rational decision to continue the hunger strike (paragraph 5), and

4   See, for example, *The Handbook of Medical Ethics*, 1984, p.44.
5   *Ibid.*

states the support of the WMA for doctors under threat for their ethical behaviour (paragraph 6). The full declaration is included in the appendices to this report.

This declaration formed an important starting point for a code of ethics drafted by the Council of International Organizations of the Medical Sciences (CIOMS) at the request of the World Health Organization and adopted by the United Nations General Assembly in December 1982. The *Principles of Medical Ethics* embody similar values to those of the *Declaration of Tokyo* though, importantly, they apply also to other health personnel. They start by insisting that doctors have an obligation to provide prisoners with the same standard of care available to free citizens. They prohibit medical involvement in torture or other cruel, inhuman or degrading treatment or punishment (principle 2), and medical engagement in a professional relationship with a prisoner not intended solely "to evaluate, protect or improve their physical and mental health" (principle 3).

Principle 4 states that it is a contravention of medical ethics for health personnel, particularly physicians:

(a) to apply their knowledge and skills in order to assist in the interrogation of prisoners and detainees in a manner that may adversely affect the physical or mental health or condition of such prisoners or detainees or which is not in accordance with the relevant international instruments;

(b) to certify, or to participate in the certification of, the fitness of prisoners or detainees for any form of treatment or punishment that may adversely affect their physical or mental health and which is not in accordance with the relevant international instruments, or to participate in any way in the infliction of any such treatment or punishment which is not in accordance with the relevant international instruments.

The restriction of the prohibition on harmful procedures to those "not in accordance with the relevant international instruments" suggested to the Working Party that there could be some procedures or punishments in which medical participation *could* be justified within the terms of the Principles. This is particularly crucial with respect to corporal punishment and the death penalty[6]. The opinion of the UN Human Rights Committee, however, that the prohibition on cruel, inhuman and

---

6 See discussion in Rodley N. *The Treatment of Prisoners under International Law.* Oxford: Clarendon Press, 1987, chapter 12.

degrading punishment "must apply to corporal punishment"[7] indicates that this particular form of punishment *could* be prohibited under principle 2 (though there has been no definitive pronouncement on this).

The reference to the legitimacy of "evaluating"[8] the health of a prisoner (principle 3) taken together with principle 4 suggests that the UN Principles of Medical Ethics could be supposed to be neutral on the question of medical involvement in the death penalty. While it is not at all clear that the Principles were *intended* to apply to the ethics of medical participation in capital punishment there are important ethical arguments concerning such involvement which will be addressed in greater detail in chapter 6.

As a result of the persistent reports of political abuse of psychiatry in the Soviet Union in the 1970s, the World Psychiatric Association adopted a Declaration at its 1977 congress in Honolulu — the *Declaration of Hawaii* — which states the internationally-agreed values of the psychiatric profession. Of particular relevance to this report is the stricture that:

> the psychiatrist must never use his professional possibilities to violate the dignity or human rights of any individual or group .... The psychiatrist must on no account utilize the tools of his profession, once the absence of psychiatric illness has been established. If a patient or some third party demands actions contrary to scientific knowledge or ethical principles the psychiatrist must refuse to cooperate. [para.7]

Other professions have codes governing their behaviour. For example, the International Council of Nurses has adopted a number of ethical statements including several relating to human rights issues, such as the role of the nurse in the care of prisoners and detainees. This report, however, concerns itself primarily with the codes and regulations by which doctors are bound.

At a regional level, there are codes applicable in Europe — the European Principles of Medical Ethics, adopted by European medical regulatory associations and similar bodies in January 1988 — and in the

---

7 United Nations. *Report of the Human Rights Committee*. Official Records of the General Assembly, 37th Session, Supplement No.40 (A/37/40), Annex V, 1982. General Comment 7(16).

8 This word was not included in the WHO-endorsed draft principles as forwarded to the UN General Assembly in 1982. It was inserted during debate and has the effect of weakening the power of the Principles with respect to examining prisoners for punishments. See Rodley N. *The Treatment of Prisoners under International Law. Op. cit.* p.297.

Islamic world. The *Declaration of Kuwait*, adopted in Kuwait in January 1981 (1401 in the Islamic calendar) by an International Conference on Islamic Medicine, is a very detailed document which includes the following passage:

> The physician shall not permit any of his special knowledge to be used to harm, destroy or inflict damage on the body, mind or spirit, whatever the military or political issues.
> The physician's one aim shall be to offer treatment and cure to the needy, be he friend or foe.

The physician's oath, which comes at the end of the Code, pledges the doctor:

> to be, all the way, an instrument of God's mercy, extending my medical care to near and far, virtuous and sinner and friend and enemy.[9]

Underlying all of these ethical codes is the basic Hippocratic principle: *primum non nocere*, above all do not harm[10]. This was restated in a modern form by the World Medical Association in the *Declaration of Geneva*[11].

International humanitarian law

The four Geneva conventions, adopted in 1949, together with additional protocols of 1977[12] set out rules for the protection for victims of wars and contain a number of provisions relevant to the rights and responsibilities of the medical profession. For example, article 16 of Protocol I (which has been signed but not yet ratified by the UK) states that "[health personnel] shall not be compelled to perform acts or to carry out work contrary to the rules of medical ethics...". References to the prohibition on torture appear at several points throughout the

---

9 An edited version of the Declaration of Kuwait was reprinted in the *World Medical Journal*, 1982; **29**:78-80.

10 Gillon has argued that *primum non nocere* is not a value advanced by Hippocrates or the Hippocratic school (Gillon R. *Philosophical Medical Ethics*. London: Wiley, 1986, p.80). The sentiment attributed to Hippocrates is nevertheless widely accepted as a fundamental basis of medicine and is used so in this report.

11 Contained in: BMA. *Handbook of Medical Ethics. Op. cit.*

12 International Committee of the Red Cross. *The Geneva Conventions of August 12 1949.* Geneva: ICRC, 1989. 245pp. ICRC. *Protocols Additional to the Geneva Conventions of 12 August 1949.* Geneva: ICRC, 1977. 124pp.

texts. For example, article 3 common to all four conventions forbids "cruel treatment and torture" and "outrages upon dignity, in particular humiliating and degrading treatment"; article 87 of the *Geneva Convention Relative to the Treatment of Prisoners of War of August 12, 1949*, prohibits "...corporal punishment, imprisonment in premises without daylight and, in general, any form of torture or cruelty".

International human rights instruments/law

References to medical or other health personnel in international human rights instruments focus principally on the rights of the prisoner or detainee to adequate medical observation and care. However, the proscriptions they contain on torture, or other cruel, inhuman or degrading treatment or punishment — when read in conjunction with the prevailing medical ethical standards — make it clear that any medical participation in such abuses is contrary to international law.

The relevant human rights standards[13] are of the following kinds:

International treaties which are binding on governments which have ratified or acceded to them:

- The International Covenant on Civil and Political Rights (adopted in 1966 and under whose terms the UN Human Rights Committee was established)
- The United Nations Convention Against Torture and other Cruel, Inhuman or Degrading Treatment or Punishment (adopted 1985)

International declarations and principles which are adopted in the UN General Assembly by consensus and which have significant moral force:

- United Nations Body of Principles for the Protection of All Persons Under any Form of Detention or Imprisonment (1988)

---

13 Human rights standards and their application are discussed in: Amnesty International. *Summary of Selected International Procedures and Bodies Dealing with Human Rights Matters.* AI Index: IOR 30/01/89, August 1989. Details of the ratification of human rights conventions by the UK government are given in appendix 10 of this report. Where countries refuse to ratify a convention they are not bound by its provisions. Nevertheless the standards embodied in the convention represent an internationally-accepted goal or standard since they come into being by agreement at the UN. Indeed, torture and cruel, inhuman or degrading treatment or punishment is understood to be prohibited under international law regardless of a country's position on particular treaties. See: Rodley N. *Op. cit.* pp.59-69.

- United Nations Standard Minimum Rules for the Treatment of Prisoners (adopted 1955)
- United Nations Declaration on the Protection of All Persons from Being Subjected to Torture and Other Cruel, Inhuman or Degrading Treatment or Punishment (adopted 1975)
- Principles for the Protection of Persons with Mental Illness and for the Improvement of Mental Health Care (adopted 1991)[14]

Regional Treaties (which are binding) and Principles (which are guiding) include:

- European Convention for the Protection of Human Rights and Fundamental Freedoms (adopted 1950)
- European Convention for the Prevention of Torture and Inhuman or Degrading Treatment or Punishment. Under this convention which came into force on 1 February 1989, a committee of experts was established with powers to visit all places of detention and imprisonment under the jurisdiction of States Parties to the Convention[15].
- European Prison Rules. These are a revision of the Standard Minimum Rules for the Treatment of Prisoners intended to guide European standards. They were adopted in 1987[16].
- Declaration of Madrid. Gives recommendations adopted by the Standing Committee of Doctors of the European Communities in 1989 regarding activities covered by the Declaration of Tokyo.

The Prison Rules are guiding while the two Conventions are binding on those governments which ratify them. The Rules make specific reference to prison medical services and the accompanying explanatory memorandum states clearly what should be regarded as "immutable" principles.

---

14 UN Document E/CN.4/1991/39, 1991.

15 The European Committee for the Prevention of Torture and Inhuman or Degrading Treatment or Punishment. For background to the Convention and working procedures see: Cassese A. A new approach to human rights: the European Convention for the Prevention of Torture. *American Journal of International Law*, 1989, **83**:128.

16 Council of Europe. *European Prison Rules*. Recommendation No. R (87) 3 adopted by the Committee of Ministers of the Council of Europe on 12 February 1987, and Explanatory Memorandum. Strasbourg, 1987.

These are that the medical officers and their staff have a primary responsibility for the medical care of the prisoners in their charge; that medical treatment and decisions should be made on professional advice and solely in the interests of the health and well-being of the patients. For prison management and administration, any executive decision that overrides or conflicts with a medical view should be reported to a higher authority and should be susceptible to review.[17]

In addition to these European standards there are regional treaties and principles in Africa and the Americas. The African Charter on Human and Peoples' Rights (adopted 1981) prohibits "all forms of exploitation and degradation of man ... particularly torture, [and] cruel, inhuman or degrading treatment and punishment". The treaty came into force on 21 October 1986 and is supervised by a Commission[18] comprising 11 members elected by governments of the states belonging to the Organization of African Unity (OAU). The commission members serve six-year terms and act in their personal capacity.

Quite apart from the legal and moral case against human rights violations, it is clear that internationally, regionally and nationally there are many specific standards and laws unambiguously proscribing medical involvement in a range of human rights abuses. The Working Party therefore felt that the standards by which to judge the human rights violations considered in this report were, by and large, adequate. Where there are remaining ambiguities or uncertainties, these will be discussed as they arise.

What was less clear was the commitment to the enforcing of, or monitoring the compliance with, all these standards. With respect to the medical codes, at a national level there are discrepancies in the enthusiasm with which those who infringe ethical standards are investigated and disciplined if found guilty of gross breaches. In some cases the medical associations charged with controlling medical ethics are themselves in the hands of military or government agents, sometimes because the legitimate leaders of the association are under threat or actually in prison. This raises the important question of the role of free associations such as the BMA in the face of this reality — a theme to which we will return later in this report.

---

17 *Ibid.* p.44.

18 The African Commission on Human and Peoples' Rights. A description of the work of the Commission can be found in: Amnesty International. *Protecting Human Rights: international procedures and how to use them. The Organization of African Unity and Human Rights.* AI Index: IOR 63/01/91, July 1991.

The major enforceable human rights instruments — those which governments have publicly committed themselves to uphold — are the benchmarks for assessing the role of the international standard in protecting human rights. The effectiveness of these conventions and declarations is mixed, with some countries either disregarding the terms of the conventions or else failing to ratify them and therefore declining to be bound by their provisions. However, they do have two major virtues. Firstly, those standards requiring regular reports to the United Nations allow for periodic and public scrutiny of a country's human rights performance and allow for the international community to call such countries to account for their behaviour.

Secondly, both binding and non-binding human rights standards offer a yardstick with which to measure a country's human rights performance. Therefore, despite the unevenness in compliance with international law, the pressure to respect human rights through, for example, the political embarrassment occasioned by annual exposure before the UN Human Rights Commission, is sufficient to suggest that continuing pressure should be put on those governments which have not yet ratified the conventions to do so.

Chapter 3

Assessing the evidence: the analytical framework

There are a number of methodological difficulties in assessing the nature and level of medical involvement in human rights abuses around the world. In particular, there are problems of definitions and comparability of data, lack of geographical balance in availability of information, difficulties in the verification of the available evidence and in the assessment of the scale of the problem both within a particular country and globally. This last problem appears to be particularly acute since torture is frequently carried out in secret and is denied by governments. This chapter sets out the analytical framework in which the Working Party undertook its analysis.

The definition of torture used in this report was given in the Preface (see p.xvi). Torture is a form of cruel, inhuman or degrading treatment or punishment, albeit a particularly serious form. For this reason, the Working Party did not attempt to make a rigorous distinction between torture in the strict sense of the word and other violations which might fall short of torture but which are nevertheless cruel, inhuman or degrading[1]. In fact, the applicable ethical standards prohibit medical involvement in both. This has avoided any possible inconsistencies between data where the same behaviour might be judged by one source as torture and by another as falling short of torture and being better described as cruel, inhuman and degrading punishment.

Corporal punishments were considered a separate issue since they are judicially inflicted and are therefore subject to judicial regulation. They differ from torture, therefore, not only in their legality under certain national laws but, arguably, also in their goals which are essentially penal and intended to control illegal behaviour.

---

1 For a discussion of the distinction between "torture" and "cruel, inhuman or degrading treatment or punishment", see: Rodley N. *The Treatment of Prisoners under International Law*. Oxford: OUP, 1987, chapter 3.

Torture: the scale of the problem

Several non-governmental and inter-governmental organizations document torture. One organization which is regarded as providing an authoritative assessment of the occurrence of torture world-wide is the human rights organization Amnesty International (AI). In its 1984 report on torture, AI concluded that the abuse was systematically or episodically practised in 66 countries and set out details of the available evidence[2]. In a further 32 countries, credible allegations of isolated incidents of torture had been reported to the organization. In AI's most recent annual reports, torture was reported to have occurred in around 65 countries[3].

There were, however, some countries where there is inadequate information available because of the closed nature of the country. North Korea represents such a case. Similarly, other international investigative bodies have been denied access to some regions or countries. Although some authorities attempt to bar investigations by representatives of large international bodies, smaller unofficial organizations may gain access. This happened in Kashmir in 1991, when a member of the European Parliament was refused admission but two doctors representing Physicians for Human Rights (UK) visited the Kashmiri capital Srinagar and reported, *inter alia*, on torture and deaths in detention[4]. Nevertheless, it appears very probable that some regimes which practice torture and other human rights abuses successfully prevent investigators from entering the territories where they operate. In certain countries, such as China, all agencies may have difficulties monitoring events because of the sheer size and communication problems involved.

A further factor to be taken into account in assessing the scale of torture is the delay between the act of torture and the fact of the torture becoming known. Torture often takes place in secrecy. Victims of torture can be held isolated for prolonged periods, the evidence only coming to light when the prisoner is released. Even then, the repressive nature of the government may mean that news about the torture is not published or distributed. Alternatively, the prisoner may not want the story of torture to become public knowledge because of a sense of

---

2 Amnesty International. *Torture in the Eighties*. London: AI, 1984.

3 *Amnesty International Report 1991*. London: AI, 1991.

4 Physicians for Human Rights (UK). *Kashmir 1991: Health Consequences of the Civil Unrest and the Police and Military Action*. London: PHR(UK), undated [1991].

shame, to avoid further personal risk or to prevent harm coming to his or her family. Even where torture allegations are made in court, the victim may not be able, or want, to identify the perpetrators. For example, a Brazilian journalist testified in a court in 1973 that, "in response to questions from the lieutenant-colonel [president of the military court]...she might be able to recognize her aggressors, but that she would rather not do it, because one of them threatened to kill her, saying that he would run her over with his car. She added that to this day she is terrified by what she saw and heard...".[5].

For these reasons amongst others, human rights organizations such as the Association of Christians for the Abolition of Torture, the International Federation of Human Rights, the International Organization against Torture/SOS-Torture, Human Rights Watch and Amnesty International eschew quantitative measures of torture nationally and globally. However, a reading of these organizations' reports (and particularly the detailed country entries of the annual Amnesty International reports) permits one to conclude whether the torture, as reported, represented isolated instances or a more systematic practice.

While levels of torture and other abuses within an individual country can only be assessed, at best, in a crude semi-quantitative fashion, there is more known about the practice of torture today than in any earlier epoch due to the courageous activities of individuals and human rights groups and the systematic work of international monitoring agencies.

However, with regard to medical involvement in torture and other abuses, a balanced picture is even more difficult to obtain. In addition to the inherent problem of assessing levels of torture itself, there is a serious problem in establishing:

- whether the absence of reports of encounters with medical personnel in the testimony of victims of torture really means that doctors were not present during their detention or merely that they did not think it a significant factor to recall
- whether the putative medical personnel were indeed doctors, other health professionals or unqualified prison personnel (since the "doctors" involved will not advertise their qualifications)
- whether the behaviour attributed to the medical personnel actually happened and, if it did, whether it was unethical.

---

5 Court records cited in *Torture in Brazil. A report by the Archdiocese of São Paulo*. (Trans. J. Wright; Ed. J. Casson). New York: Vintage, 1986, p.185.

With respect to the first point, it is not possible to know whether the absence of testimony of medical involvement indicates the absence of such involvement or merely a failure to report it. Certainly it is possible that to some victims of torture:

> the doctor was only one of many abusers and may not have appeared a significant figure.... [Moreover] in some cases the detainee may have been blindfold or unable for other reasons to determine whether there was a doctor present; in other cases, the detainee may not have been able to judge whether a person carrying out a medical examination was indeed a doctor[6].

Again with respect to the medical qualifications of those thought by prisoners to be doctors, it appears to be generally necessary to rely on patterns of evidence rather than on individual and isolated testimony: repeated testimonies of the presence of a doctor at interrogations in a particular detention centre — each contributing a particular insight into the "doctor's" behaviour — can add up to compelling evidence of medical participation. In some cases, the demeanour and techniques of "doctors" during examinations is strongly suggestive to the prisoner that they are in medical hands. For example, one of the former prisoners examined by an Amnesty International medical delegation to Chile sought:

> to discover whether it really was a doctor examining him [and] told him he had *situs inversus* [i.e. the position of body organs is the reverse of normal] and that it was very serious. The doctor assured him that it was not and gave a correct account of the condition[7].

In other cases, doctors who themselves were detainees were able to make judgements about the person playing the medical role. For example, Dr Sergio Arroyo, a Chilean doctor arrested in May 1981, told Amnesty International medical delegates that he was convinced that the person who examined him was a doctor because of the way medical questions were put and the technique of physical examination[8].

A third situation in which an allegation of medical involvement can be validated is where the victim knows the doctor, either personally or through family connections. For example, the Argentinean journalist

---

6 Amnesty International. *Involvement of medical personnel in abuses against detainees and prisoners.* AI Index: ACT 75/08/90, November 1990.

7 *Chile: Evidence of torture.* London: Amnesty International, 1983, p.48.

8 *Ibid.* p.60.

Jacobo Timerman recalled in a memoir of his prison experience an encounter with a prison doctor following his torture.

> He examines my gums and advises me not to worry, I'm in perfect health. He tells me that he's proud of the way I withstood it all. Some people die on their torturers, without a decision being made to kill them; this is regarded as a professional failure. He indicates that I was once a friend of his father's, also a police doctor. His features do seem familiar. I mention his father's name; this is indeed the son. He assures me that I'm not going to be killed. I tell him that I haven't been tortured for two days and he's pleased.[9]

However, while we can be confident that many reports of medical involvement do refer to doctors, we have to accept that some reports may in fact implicate nurses, paramedics or even guards with some medical awareness. Assessing whether the behaviour allegedly perpetrated by the "doctor" really took place is most easily assessed when there is a pattern of medical contact with prisoners in a place where human rights violations are documented. It is then possible to assess each new allegation in the light of existing knowledge. Isolated allegations must be evaluated by normal methods of assessing evidence: is the story internally consistent? does it fit in with what is already known of the country? is the witness a credible person? are there any evident ulterior motives for the witness's testimony? Having established whether or not the reported incident is likely to have happened, the evaluation of the ethics of the behaviour of the doctor in question remains. This will be addressed in the next chapter.

While direct examination of primary evidence is always desirable, the Working Party was, for the most part, forced to rely on the evaluations of available evidence made by others: human rights sources who had collected evidence, medical organizations which had investigated aspects of the subject, and medical associations which had undertaken investigations of torture allegations made against their members or others working in their country. In addition to such secondary sources, the Working Party was able to interview in person a limited number of witnesses concerning the above issues.

---

9   Timerman J. *Prisoner without a Name, Cell without a Number*. (trans. T Talbot.) London: Weidenfeld and Nicolson, 1981, p.54.

Medical involvement in torture

There have been very few attempts to assess levels of medical involvement in human rights violations. Where judicial investigations of war crimes, torture or other human rights violations have been carried out there have been relatively few doctors prosecuted. For example, following the trials which took place in the immediate post-War period, some 20 doctors were tried for war crimes — only a fraction of the 350 doctors thought to have actively worked in the Nazi "medical programme"[10]. Following the documentation of medical atrocities carried out in Japan there were no prosecutions of doctors involved. The reasons were given in a report of a sub-committee of a US State-War-Navy [Departments'] Coordinating Committee which evaluated prosecution policy in 1947:

> ...c) The value to the US of Japanese BW [biological warfare] data is of such importance to national security as to far outweigh the value accruing from 'war crimes' prosecution. d) In the interests of national security it would not be advisable to make this information available to other nations as would be the case in the event of a 'war crimes' trial of Japanese BW experts. e) The BW information obtained from Japanese sources should be retained in Intelligence channels and should not be employed as 'war crimes' evidence.[11]

In more recent times the same pattern is evident. The 1975 trials which followed the fall from power of the Greek colonels in the previous year saw the conviction of only one doctor, Dr Dimitrios Kofas, who was sentenced to seven years' imprisonment[12]. Similarly, in Argentina only one doctor was convicted of participation in torture following the return to democracy in 1983[13]. Prosecutions, therefore, can be regarded as

---

10 Mitscherlich A, Mielke F. *The Death Doctors*. London: Elek, 1962, p.17; Proctor R. *Racial Hygiene: Medicine Under the Nazis*. Cambridge MA: Harvard University Press, 1989. The number of doctors "involved" in Nazi medicine clearly depends on how involvement is defined. The numbers tolerating abuses or knowing of them is likely to have been significantly larger.

11 Cited in Williams P, Wallace D. *Unit 731*. London: Grafton, 1990, p.314.

12 *Torture in Greece: the First Torturer's Trial 1975*. London: Amnesty International, 1977.

13 This doctor, Dr Antonio Berges, was sentenced on 2 December 1986 to six years' imprisonment on two counts of torture but was released from prison in June 1987 under the terms of the Law of Due Obedience (*Ley de obediencia debida*) which absolved all but the highest ranking officers of human rights crimes. See Amnesty International. *Argentina: Doctor convicted of torture released under "due*

a poor indicator of the scale of the phenomenon, seriously under-estimating its occurrence.

Throughout 1990 and 1991, allegations were widely reported concerning medical participation in a variety of punitive measures and human rights abuses in the former German Democratic Republic (GDR)[14]. These reports demonstrate some of the difficulties in making a realistic assessment of the scale of medical involvement in a given situation. To some extent, they also encapsulate the problems of attempting to make value judgements of behaviour occurring in a closed society where different moral norms and social pressures pertain from those which are widely accepted in our own situation.

To briefly summarise the background, the secret police (Stasi) formed an all pervasive element in the regime which governed East German life for 40 years. It has been estimated that between 150,000 and 500,000 citizens acted as Stasi informers and when the Ministry of State Security was raided in January 1990, records showed that around 90,000 people were on the Stasi payroll. The atmosphere of secrecy was such that, even within families and close relationships, individuals worked for the Stasi without this fact being known. These people were drawn from all walks of life and included a significant number of doctors. The Stasi function of doctors would be likely to have ranged from serious collaboration encompassing harm or potential harm to patients to the ubiquitous practice of passing on information of varying importance about the "inner enemy" or about colleagues. In the range of serious offenses, doctors are alleged to have been involved in psychiatric abuse for political purposes, potentially dangerous experimentation on patients and gravely improper treatment of patients brought to serve as organ donors to the Charité hospital in East Berlin, where 30 doctors are said to have been Stasi employees[15]. It is, as yet, too early to report on the nature and scale of such abuses.

Various attempts have been made to assess the scale of medical involvement and some estimates have been made suggesting that as

---

obedience" law. AI Index: AMR 13/10/87, 17 December 1987. Some doctors were named in publications as human rights violators but were never punished. Given the scale of human rights violations in Argentina, the number of prosecutions in general was very low.

14 See the series of articles by Annette Tuffs on Germany: Psychiatry in the East. *Lancet*, 1990; **335**:1392; Investigation of psychiatric abuse. *Lancet*, 1990; **336**:1434-5; Horror hospital. *Lancet*, 1991; **338**:624. Doctor spies. *Lancet*, 1992; **339**:356. See also: *Der Spiegel*, 26 August 1991 and 2 September 1991.

15 *Lancet*, 1991; **338**:624.

many as 50 percent of East German doctors were involved to some degree[16] with the Stasi. Such a figure is not very illuminating, however, considering the wide range of practices which might be considered as "involvement". In 1991 the Berlin Senate distributed questionnaires to all health workers in municipal and state-run hospitals to determine each individual's relationship to the Stasi, since Federal law prohibited the employment of former Stasi employees in state facilities. Those who admitted Stasi involvement were dismissed. These tended to be employees in the lower echelons, as people with more influence were able to utilise the time between the fall of the Berlin wall in November 1989 and the seizing of Stasi headquarters in January 1990 to try to destroy compromising files about themselves.

Nevertheless, of 5000 medical staff employed at the Charité hospital, about 20 doctors including 15 professors were dismissed in July and August 1991 when Stasi contracts identifying them were discovered. Those allegedly involved in organ transplantation misconduct may face criminal charges. The Berlin Chamber of Physicians also attempted to bring 14 of its members before a professional disciplinary tribunal (*Ehrengericht*) to prevent them from working as doctors. This move has been criticised by some on grounds of arbitrariness as the doctors were not given a hearing or leave to appeal. Others feel that more action is needed but there have been considerable problems in conducting fact-finding investigations. For example, a committee ordered by the GDR Parliament in March 1990, investigated the abuse of psychiatry, principally at the Waldheim clinic in Hochweitzschen, whose director was a Stasi member. The preliminary Waldheim report, published in 1990, indicated that some East German psychiatrists appointed to a second investigative committee were themselves involved in the original abuses[17].

In a presentation cited above, Dr Claudia Malzfeldt pointed to a reluctance on many levels of society in the united Germany to acknowledge what had occurred in the GDR:

> We [in West Germany] could have known more but we were not really interested in knowing details. We could not accept the fact of unlawfulness and violence, right next to us in Europe. Now, most people from the GDR do not want to hear any more. They can't stand the pain

---

16 Malzfeldt C. Paper given at symposium on health and human rights in Eastern Europe. Amsterdam: Johannes Wier Stichting, 1 November 1991.

17 Tuffs A. Germany: Investigation of psychiatric abuse. *Lancet*, 1990; **336**:1434-5.

any more or the confrontation with the truth. Also hundreds of thousands of people definitely do fear being uncovered as having been collaborators.

Some indication of participation in particular countries can be gleaned from investigations carried out by medical associations or other bodies. For example, the Uruguayan National Commission of Medical Ethics reported having investigated more than 80 doctors against whom allegations of involvement in human rights violations were received. However, the Commission was only able to sustain charges against a small number, probably in part because of the stringent evidential requirement of their judicial process[18]. Similarly, persistent reports of medical involvement in the 1970s and 1980s in Chile have been investigated by the *Colegio Médico de Chile*; only a small number of doctors have been disciplined. In Turkey, the medical association has investigated torture allegations arising during the period of military government but could not find proof that any physician participated or helped in torture. Three physicians were suspended for six months for false certification and lawyers submitted the names of a further 32 physicians to the association for investigation[19].

In Brazil and Argentina, commissions of enquiry into torture during the periods of military rule presented evidence of medical involvement in human rights violations. The Brazilian report, *Brasil: Nunca Mais* (Brazil: Never Again), prepared under the sponsorship of the Catholic Church, drew on official court records to document the systematic use of torture during the majority of the period of military rule, 1964-79. Testimonies given to the court contained references to doctors examining, reviving, treating and observing prisoners during and after torture; in many cases they provided false or inadequate medical certificates. The report names around a dozen doctors alleged to have prepared false medical certificates[20]. The Argentinian report which, significantly, bore a similar title — *Nunca Más* — was the work of the National Commission on Disappeared People. It also referred to

18 For example, the National Commission of Medical Ethics would not proceed on the basis of existing published testimonies implicating doctors but rather required that individuals personally submit new signed testimonies. Evidence given to the Working Party by Dr Gregorio Martirena, *Federación Médica del Interior*, Uruguay, June 1990. See also: Martirena G. *La Tortura y los Médicos*. Montevideo: Ediciones de la Banda Oriental, 1988.

19 Lök V. Turkish doctors act against their torturer colleagues. *International Newsletter on Treatment and Rehabilitation of Torture Victims*, 1989, **1**:5-6.

20 *Torture in Brazil*, p.37.

evidence of medical collaboration in human rights violations though the nature of repression in Argentina — disappearance and killing — was such that evidence of medical assistance was likely to be harder to obtain[21].

The medical literature does not help in assessing the level of medical participation. Rasmussen[22], for example, who presented evidence that 41 of 200 victims of torture comprising his study had reported that medical personnel had been involved in their torture, did not draw any general conclusions about the wider scale of torture. Neither did Allodi and Cowgill who reported that 19 out of the 41 subjects of their study had seen or been treated by 21 doctors during their imprisonment[23]. However, using a wide definition of medical involvement, Vesti found that 29 of his study population of 42 had experienced medical participation in their torture and suggested that it might be a widespread phenomenon in all parts of the world[24].

In fact, attempting to quantify medical involvement immediately throws up the problem of defining what is meant by "quantity" in this context. For example, a single doctor who monitored every prisoner tortured in a particular prison or detention centre would represent an involvement level of 100% from the point of view of the prisoners. However, as a percentage of the medical profession in the state, a single doctor could represent a minuscule fraction. On the other hand, if scores or hundreds of doctors were involved in the torture of a relatively small number of prisoners, the picture would be reversed: a higher percentage of doctors would be involved but from the prisoner's perspective there would be a limited level of medical involvement. This suggests that a "percent involvement" figure is likely to be a very rough and ready measure.

Taking into account all these unavoidable limitations, the Working Party felt that it would not be possible to draw any firm conclusions

---

21 *Nunca Más*. London: Faber and Faber, 1986.

22 Rasmussen OV. *Medical Aspects of Torture*. Supplement 1 of *Danish Medical Bulletin*, 1990; 37:88pp.

23 Allodi F, Cowgill G. Ethical and psychiatric aspects of torture: a Canadian study. *Canadian Journal of Psychiatry*, 1982, 27:98-102.

24 Vesti P. Extreme man-made stress and anti-therapy: doctors as collaborators in torture. *Danish Medical Bulletin*, 1990; 37:466-8. Dr Vesti defined medical involvement as occurring "when [doctors] evaluate and/or treat the victim at the request of the authorities. They are also considered to be involved actively when they are simply present in the room or in the place of detention." (This is wider than the definition used by the Working Party for this report — see p.34 below.)

about "quantities" of torture or medical involvement and that, at best, it would only be able to draw conclusions about its existence and its significance; that is, whether the medical profession should regard the problem as an important or minor ethical issue. The past history of child abuse shows that the fact that such abuses are hidden, unrecognized, or "unmeasurable" by society does not make them any the less a social and medical problem and, as later chapters will show, the Working Party found the involvement of doctors in torture to be a significant ethical issue.

Abuse of psychiatry

The abuse of psychiatry for political purposes can embody elements of torture, or of other cruel, inhuman or degrading treatment: involuntary and painful administration of unnecessary medication; beatings and physical restraint; humiliation and degradation; indefinite separation from loved ones. However, where psychiatric abuse differs significantly from other forms of political abuse is in the framework in which it is carried out. Firstly, the laws which allow compulsory committal to a psychiatric hospital are intended for the patient's good; secondly, the agents of the abuse are doctors and other "medical staff"[25] who may or may not believe that they are acting according to the patient's medical needs; thirdly, the political thoughts of the victim may be seen, not only as subversive and dangerous, but as a sign of illness; fourthly, the procedures used to enforce committal may well not permit recourse to the law since legal appeal mechanisms in cases of mental illness have historically been weak. Because of these differences, the Working Party felt it important to look at psychiatric abuse separately.

In assessing the evidence of psychiatric abuse, the Working Party relied in great measure on the documentation available from organizations such as the International Association on the Political Use of Psychiatry, different psychiatric associations, including the Royal College of Psychiatrists, and human rights bodies such as Helsinki Watch and Amnesty International. Evidence from a US delegation of psychiatrists which visited the USSR in 1989 and a World Psychiatric Association delegation in June 1991, were reviewed, as well as personal testimony from a Soviet psychiatrist and former prisoner, Semyon Gluzman, who gave evidence in person in June 1990. In addition, recent

---

25 As noted above (p.24), not all those who look like medical staff are necessarily what they seem.

criticisms of political abuses of psychiatry from within the USSR[26] have helped to inform the deliberations of the Working Party. These acknowledgements of the failure of the law to protect Soviet citizens appear to confirm the validity of much of the criticism directed towards Soviet psychiatric practice for more than two decades. Clearly recent political changes will have major implications for psychiatric practice in the various former Soviet republics.

Questions of the possible abuse of psychiatric knowledge and procedures in the practice of capital punishment will be addressed separately in chapter 6.

Corporal and capital punishments

With respect to these two forms of punishment, the information gathering and evaluation process was a little different to that applied to torture and psychiatric abuse inasmuch as both forms of punishment are legal and therefore to some extent open to scrutiny. However, although such practices are lawful in those countries where they are practised, it does not automatically follow that evidence of their occurrence is easily obtainable. For example, the USSR/CIS, Japan and Saudi Arabia among others do not publish statistics on capital punishment and evidence has to be gathered from unofficial sources. In addition, there remained certain problems similar to those encountered with compiling information on torture. Corporal punishment and capital punishment do not provoke the same level of research or campaigning as torture, and the level of basic information is less. Amnesty International appears to be the only organization systematically compiling information on the death penalty world-wide[27], while the same organization records the use of corporal punishment wherever it has been able to obtain information.

---

26 *Information Bulletin No.17*. International Association on the Political Use of Psychiatry, December 1987; Amnesty International. *USSR: Human rights in a time of change*. AI Index: EUR 46/22/89, October 1989.

27 Amnesty International. *When the State Kills*. London: AI, 1989. AI publishes a monthly death penalty bulletin. The United Nations periodically reviews the practice of capital punishment but is dependent on five-yearly reports submitted by governments. See, for example, the most recent report, *Capital punishment: Report of the Secretary-General*, Economic and Social Council: E/1990/38/Rev.1, 15 June 1990. This notes that "replies [to the UN questionnaire] were received from 55 Governments only" [p.5] limiting the analysis possible. See also: Hood R. *The Death Penalty: a World-wide Perspective*. Oxford: Clarendon Press, 1989. 182pp.

However, detailed information on death penalty procedures in countries using the punishment are not easily obtained. In some countries the execution is carried out virtually in secret. Moreover, published research on the death penalty focuses overwhelmingly on the USA and, to a lesser extent, Europe. Less than five percent of research published in the period 1979-86 dealt with developing countries[28]. A small fraction of all this research dealt with medical issues and this was focused on the USA. The Working Party had to accept therefore that there would be an inevitable bias towards the ethical dilemmas posed to doctors as experienced in the USA though some, if not most, could in principle be faced by doctors elsewhere.

Conclusion

The Working Party felt that the oral and written evidence it received, as well as the documentation with which it was provided, was substantially credible. Moreover, it was presented with adequate recognition and acknowledgement of inherent limitations to allow for an evaluation of the nature of medical involvement in the human rights violations which were the subject of the Working Party's investigation. Although the Working Party had intended to focus its enquiries on evidence of medical involvement in abuses since the publication of the 1986 BMA report, it was found during the course of investigations that such a policy was unworkable. Evidence of torture in many cases is not available for a long time after the event and the evidence reviewed by the Working Party, although much of it emanating from recently published material, nevertheless included reference to events happening as far back as the 1970s.

For the reasons outlined above, the Working Party did not feel that, in general, it was able to accurately assess the *scale* of the problem in quantitative terms. This subject will be considered in more detail in the chapters that follow.

---

28 Zvekic U, Kubo T. Main trends in research on capital punishment (1979-1986). *Revue Internationale de Droit Pénal*, 1987; **58**:533-54.

Chapter 4

Medical involvement in torture

[The prisoner] said that in June 1963, he got into a fight ... and was hit on the foot with a hoe. He had been hospitalized for three days when Mr Bruton [the superintendent] came to see him and asked what happened. Mr Bruton then had him put on a table in the prison hospital, belted down with one strap across his chest and one across his legs. The inmate doctor wired him up on the "Tucker Telephone" with one wire to his penis and another to his big toe. The telephone was cranked five or six times. [An informant] stated that this instrument was designed by Dr Rollins (former prison doctor) and consisted of an electrical generator taken from a ring-type telephone, placed in sequence with two dry cell batteries, and attached to an undressed inmate on the treatment table at the Tucker Hospital by means of one electrode to a big toe and the second electrode to the penis, at which time a crank was turned sending an electrical charge into the body of the inmate. He stated that several charges were introduced into the inmates of a duration designed to stop just short of the inmate "passing out".[1]

This passage illustrates an unambiguous story of medical involvement in torture. In this case the word "involvement" is clear. The doctor was an integral player in an episode of unacceptable and unethical violation of human rights. However, what *are* the limits which define unacceptable involvement? When does a doctor or other health worker move from being a reluctant bystander uncertain that torture has taken place and uncertain of what to do about it, if it has, to becoming an integral component of an atrocity?

The standard established by the World Medical Association — the Declaration of Tokyo — gives little scope for ambiguity on whether or not doctors should become involved in torture. It makes clear that "the doctor shall not countenance, condone or participate in the practice of torture or other forms of cruel, inhuman or degrading procedures,

---

1 Arkansas State Police, Criminal Investigations Division. *Case report: Tucker State Prison Farm, Tucker, Arkansas,* (Little Rock, Arkansas, circa September 1966). Cited by Murton T. Prison doctors. In: Visscher MB (ed.) *Humanistic Perspectives in Medical Ethics*, Buffalo: Prometheus Books, 1972, pp.248-9.

whatever the offence of which the victim is suspected, accused or guilty...". This formulation addresses itself to a spectrum of engagement by medical personnel in human rights violations which can be broken down into three phases: the preparatory phase; the execution phase; and the recovery phase. Medical personnel can and do play a role in each of these phases.

For the purposes of this report, the Working Party considered that medical involvement or participation in torture might arise when a doctor was involved in a relationship with a prisoner:

- immediately before, during, or after torture
- without the free consent of the prisoner
- with either the prisoner or the doctor not being free to identify themselves (or with the doctor refusing to be identified)
- where the doctor acted in the interests of persons other than the prisoner

In addition, medical participation was considered to have occurred when a doctor undertook any examination, certification or forensic assessment of a tortured prisoner or ex-prisoner (or remains of a prisoner), in which he or she failed to record a prisoner's complaints or to record signs of ill-treatment or other marks or injuries relevant to the prisoner's case. In some cases, the issuing of false certificates or forensic reports, while initially obstructing the search for the truth, subsequently provided the rare solid documentary evidence of medical collaboration in torture.

The medical associations which have carried out investigations have described their own definitions of participation. The National Commission of Medical Ethics, established in Uruguay in 1985 to investigate allegations of violations by doctors, outlined its concerns as follows: passing clinical records to the military; drafting reports or certificates which concealed torture; failure to give adequate medical care; injurious delay in referring prisoners to intensive care; participation in interrogation and torture; design of a prison regime intended to physically and psychologically destroy prisoners[2].

The Chilean Medical Association summarized the participation of doctors in torture as follows:

1. Evaluating the victim's capacity to withstand torture.
2. Supervising torture through the provision of medical treatment if complications occur.

---

2   Document 13. Seminar on "Physicians, ethics and torture", Montevideo, Uruguay, 9-12 December 1987.

3. Providing professional knowledge and skills to the torturer.
4. Falsifying or deliberately omitting medical information when issuing health certificates or autopsy reports.
5. Providing medical assistance within the torture system without either denouncing torture or resigning from such work.
6. Administering torture by directly participating in it.
7. Remaining silent in spite of the knowledge that abuses have taken place.[3]

Both these associations provided important evidence to the Working Party, through correspondence, verbal evidence and documentation.

Outside the actual torture itself, doctors seeing victims of torture can act in good or bad faith — a differentiation which will be discussed below.

Why do doctors get involved?

Few of the available studies on the motivation and behaviour of torturers have looked specifically at what motivates doctors who assist in the torture of prisoners. The most detailed is Lifton's study of Nazi doctors[4]; others have looked at training and motivation of torturers in general. The available evidence suggests that those who participate in torture (including those with medical qualifications) are not exceptional or uniquely evil persons[5]. They could be, in the words of one young Greek man prosecuted for acts related to torture, "your neighbour's son"[6].

Studies of the last decade on the psychology of the torturer suggest that certain individual psychosocial characteristics and underlying cultural and political factors contribute to the recruitment of particular

---

3 See: The Participation of Physicians in Torture. A report of the Chilean Medical Association, 1986. In: Stover E. *The Open Secret: Torture and the Medical Profession in Chile*. Washington DC: American Association for the Advancement of Science, 1987, p.75.

4 Lifton RJ. *The Nazi Doctors: The Psychology of Medical Killing*. London: Papermac, 1986.

5 Milgram S. *Obedience to Authority*. London: Tavistock, 1974.

6 Testimony given by Alexandros Lavranos, prosecuted in 1975 for torture-related crimes carried out during the period of military rule in Greece. He was acquitted by the court. See: Amnesty International. *Torture in Greece: The First Torturers' Trial 1975*. London: AI Publications, 1977, p.42. The phrase was used as the title of a film on the training of Greek torturers. *Your Neighbour's Son: The Making of a Torturer*. Producer: Ebbe Preisler Film, Copenhagen; Directors: Jørgen Flindt Pedersen and Erik Stephensen. Denmark, 1982.

individuals (usually via incorporation into the military) into a torture squad. Gibson and Haritos-Fatouros[7], for example, have examined the training and development of Greek torturers during the period 1967-74. They focused particularly on the training of military personnel and documented the various techniques and military recruitment and training procedures which facilitated the development of an obedient torturer.

Staub, in a lengthy review of the psychology of torture[8], suggested a number of mechanisms by which a person could become able to carry out terrible acts which would seem at first sight to be incompatible with the individual's moral beliefs. By looking at the practice of torture at three levels — individual psychology, sub-group and group processes, and cultural and historical societal processes — he sets out to present an understanding of the underlying motivation, development and psychology of the torturer. His analysis can only be touched on here, but it draws together elements such as:

Discrimination against and labelling or devaluing of a victim group. In some states particular minorities are identified as the scape-goats for societal problems. Negative stereotypes gain currency and the labelled group is transformed into an "out-group" which lacks the basic human characteristics which binds the members of the majority into a cohesive whole.

Training. The focus of military training is obedience to orders so that a military goal can be achieved. Studies based on experiments such as those of Zimbardo and associates[9], as well as on observations of the development of torture in the Greek army, suggest that training and "learning by doing" play a significant part in effecting a capacity for torture in an individual.

Existence of a tendency to blame the victim (a "just-world view"). Staub suggests that witnessing the suffering of others can induce in the observer a belief that the affected individual must be responsible in some way for his or her fate — that in a just world, people get what

---

7   Gibson J, Haritos-Fatouros M. The education of a torturer. *Psychology Today*, 1986, **20**:50-58; Gibson J. Factors contributing to the creation of a torturer. In: *Psychology and Torture* (ed. P. Suedfeld). New York: Hemisphere, 1990, pp.77-88. Haritos-Fatouros M. The official torturer: a learning model for obedience to the authority of violence. *Journal of Applied Social Psychology*, 1988, **18**:1107-20.

8   Staub E. The psychology and culture of torture and torturers. In: *Psychology and Torture. Op. cit.* pp.49-76.

9   Zimbardo PG, Haney C, Banks WC, Jaffe D. The psychology of imprisonment: privation, power and pathology. In: Zubin Z (ed.) *Doing Unto Others*. Englewood Cliffs: Prentice Hall, 1974.

they deserve. Thus those who are victimised must in some way deserve their treatment.

Other elements of Staub's analysis include: the existence of an ideology tolerant of torture, individual obedience to a repressive authority, a system of rewards for those engaged in torture, as well as cultural and societal processes which embody most of these elements. Staub illustrates his thesis with examples from Nazi Germany, Argentina and other countries. He suggests that:

> Although a majority of people can probably be led to torture others, they require different degrees of pressure — the threats of force, motivation arising from culture and life conditions, or the promise of rewards. When a whole society moves along the continuum of destruction, as individuals are re-socialized, the mistreatment and destruction of others become easier and more possible for many people.[10]

With regard to the medical role, Lifton's seminal study on Nazi doctors proposed mechanisms by which doctors could undertake such appalling breaches of medical ethics as assisting in the "euthanasia" of the mentally ill and handicapped, and medical experimentation on prisoners. Lifton suggested that a psychological process he called "doubling" was brought into play to allow the doctor to manage two value systems which were mutually contradictory. It allowed the "division of the self into two functioning wholes, so that the part-self acts as an entire self".

> Doubling is an active psychological process, a means of *adaptation to extremity*. ... The adaptation requires a dissolving of 'psychic glue' as an alternative to a radical breakdown of the self. In Auschwitz, the pattern was established under the duress of the individual doctor's transition period. At that time the Nazi doctor experienced his own death anxiety as well as such death equivalents as fear of disintegration, separation and stasis. He needed a functional Auschwitz self to still his anxiety. And that Auschwitz self had to assume hegemony on an everyday basis, reducing expressions of the prior self to odd moments and to contacts with family and friends outside the camp. Nor did most Nazi doctors resist that usurpation as long as they remained in the camp. Rather they welcomed it as the only means of psychological function. If an environment is sufficiently extreme, and one chooses to remain in it, one may be able to do so *only* by means of doubling.[11]

---

10 Staub. *Op. cit.* p.71.

11 Lifton RJ. *The Nazi Doctors: Medical Killing and the Psychology of Genocide*. London: Papermac, 1987, p.418.

Amnesty International suggested that the motivation of medical personnel who assist in torture can be attributed to one or more of the following[12]:

Identification with the cause of the torturers, due either to an absorption of the torturers' values or a pre-existing sympathy with the ruling ideology. A Uruguayan psychiatrist interviewed by Bloche told him "the war [against subversion] continued inside the prison. Day after day, rule after rule, were part of a grand design to make [the prisoners] suffer psychologically"[13].

Fear of the consequences of refusing to cooperate: This may particularly press on those young doctors who are conscripted into military service and who are subject to military discipline. As a former Chilean army doctor who gave evidence to the Working Party described, overt threats could be made to those who refused to co-operate in abuses of human rights:

> ..gradually and slowly they tried to persuade me or even force me to get involved in sinister and immoral activities. I rejected that at all times. ...
> The commanding officer...summoned me one day and said, "Either you conform to the principle of military activities, or you are going to have a pretty rough time." That developed into an argument, and he threatened me with a pistol, put a pistol in my face and said, "I could kill you if I wanted to and get away with it."[14]

This seemed to confirm testimony of a Chilean ex-military doctor cited in a report of the American Association for the Advancement of Science:

> ...we knew of others in the military, including physicians, who were involved [in torture]. Some of them collaborated because they were ordered to and because they were afraid of what might happen if they refused. In my case, I was sent on two occasions to a detention camp to treat prisoners who had been tortured. The experience troubled me so much, I began planning a way out of the service....[15]

---

12 Amnesty International. *Involvement of medical personnel in abuses against detainees and prisoners*. AI Index: ACT 75/08/90, November 1990.

13 Bloche MG. *Uruguay's Military Physicians: Cogs in a System of State Terror.* Washington: AAAS, 1987, p.15.

14 Oral evidence to the Working Party, June, 1990. Name of witness withheld.

15 Cited in Stover E. *The Open Secret: Torture and the Medical Profession in Chile. Op. cit.* p.27.

The other side of this coin is that there are undoubted advantages to "not rocking the boat", at least to the extent of not provoking strained relations with military colleagues and possibly guaranteeing a better career.

"Bureaucratization" of the medical role: For some doctors, medicine may be seen as, or may progressively acquire the character of, a technical process depending on professional skills but not requiring a moral framework (or perhaps a *different* moral framework to that generally accepted). In September 1990, a Brazilian former forensic doctor, Harry Shibata, testified at a hearing into the fate of numerous "disappeared" people whose remains were uncovered in a mass grave on the outskirts of São Paulo. Part of his testimony illustrated this view of the doctor as technician. On being asked why none of the Medicolegal Institute's autopsy reports during the military rule period mentioned torture he replied:

> Our [forensic doctor's] function was purely technical. First thing in the morning we received bodies...and we performed autopsies to establish the cause of death...our task was only to establish the medical cause of death and not the judicial cause of death....[It] is purely descriptive...all that is on the body is observed and recorded. Now, the interpretation of these lesions is something we cannot give. A haematoma could be a spontaneous haematoma or it could be a traumatic haematoma. But we just describe the haematoma.[16]

(The fact that Medicolegal Institutes are often state-supported bodies with state-paid staff almost inevitably acts to limit the independence of those staff; effectively doctors are asked by the state to investigate the possible crimes of the state: their employer.)

A Uruguayan psychiatrist who worked in Libertad prison in Uruguay during the period of military dictatorship expressed a similar desire to maintain a distance from the implications of his work, asserting that:

> I was confined to my function. I ignored some aspects and there were some aspects I didn't want to know about.... It wasn't my purpose. I am a doctor."[17]

---

16 Americas Watch *et al. The Search for Brazil's Disappeared: The Mass Grave at Dom Bosco Cemetery*. Washington: Americas Watch, March 1991, p.11. Dr Shibata was removed from the medical register by the São Paulo State Medical Council in 1980 after investigations into the torture of a politician revealed that Dr Shibata had signed a false medical certificate stating that the man showed no signs of torture.

17 Bloche MG. *Uruguay's Military Physicians: Cogs in a System of State Terror. Op. cit.* p.40.

Inadequate understanding of medical ethics. This is typified by the argument that it is better for a doctor to carry out or assist in the carrying out of a harmful punishment or torture because the doctor can minimize the pain and damage. In some cultures where infliction of corporal punishment is accepted, there is a divided view among the medical profession as to the legitimacy of medical assistance in such punishments. This will be discussed in chapter 6. The misunderstanding of the medical role in interrogation was clearly demonstrated in the UK following the use of "depth interrogation" in Northern Ireland in the early 1970s. As the 1986 BMA *Torture Report* discussed, the recommendation by the Parker Committee that "a doctor ... should be present at all times at the interrogation centre", and should be able to observe the course of oral interrogation of prisoners was rejected by both the government of the day and the BMA, and medical opposition to this role was subsequently codified in the WMA's Declaration of Tokyo in 1975[18]. Undoubtedly lack of public and professional criticism of medical involvement cannot but contribute to the perpetuation of such abuses.

How do doctors get involved?

Doctors and other medical personnel can get involved in serious violations of human rights at any point in the process. While doctors are not trained in a culture of strict obedience as are military personnel, some doctors work within a milieu where security considerations take high priority. Those who are most likely to assist in human rights abuses are the medical personnel who are directly responsible for examining and providing health care for prisoners. Some are dragged into this role by enforced conscription into military service where they can find themselves called upon to treat tortured "enemy" prisoners (whether internal opposition or external army). Even doctors who normally have no contact with detained individuals can find themselves involved with those who have been tortured or who are at risk of torture by, for example, the admission of an ill-treated detainee to a general hospital. Some doctors, who initially join the army freely, become

---

18 BMA *Torture Report*, pp.14-19. The government accepted the thrust of the minority report included in the report of the Parker Committee. *Report of the Committee of Privy Counsellors appointed to consider authorised procedures for the interrogation of persons suspected of terrorism.* Cmnd. 4901. London: HMSO, March 1972.

entangled in activities which breach internationally accepted medical standards. This was graphically described by the Chilean witness mentioned above, who had joined the army as a young doctor just prior to the September 1973 military coup, and subsequently found himself a horrified witness to a multiple extrajudicial execution:

> I was called on one occasion to go to a seaside resort to examine some prisoners who were to be transferred to Concepción. I examined the prisoners and I felt that they were fit to travel. On the way back [to Concepción] the convoy stopped and I was told to remain in the jeep. Shortly afterwards I heard some shots, I tried to get out but they forced me back in. I then literally forced my way out. I remember this more as a nightmare. I believe that some of the people or all of the people were shot there.[19]

Although this doctor had felt shocked and believed that these executions were an outrage into which he had been drawn against his will, he knew that there was no one in authority to whom he could turn, and that he was powerless to stop similar incidents happening in the future. He attempted to discuss the subject with other young doctors in the same position but found them intimidated and unwilling to discuss it or take any action. In explaining to the Working Party what ultimately prevented him from conforming to the reluctant practice of his peers, he indicated that much had hinged on having some external advice and support. Without this, he felt he might well have lost his moral perspective and obeyed his officers. After placing himself at some risk on several occasions, his "obstinacy" led to his being dismissed from the army and subsequently he went into exile. The problem of isolation is a considerable one, since no professional machinery currently exists to provide support to doctors attempting to combat abuses of human rights in situations of serious personal risk. We will return to this important question in chapter 9.

Doctors can be activists in opposition movements, either as political figures or as doctors. It is only the latter role which is considered here[20]. Evidence of their collaboration in human rights violations is particularly difficult to obtain. By their very nature, opposition groups seek internal security and doctors would almost certainly concentrate on

---

19 Oral evidence, June 1990.

20 To analyze the actions of a figure such as Dr George Habash, the leader of the Popular Front for the Liberation of Palestine, in a medical-ethical framework seems to extend the scope of medical ethics. Such non-medical activities seem better judged within the political framework in which they occur.

providing medical services to the opposition members. However allegations of improper behaviour surface infrequently. The Lebanese doctor Aziz al-Abub has been alleged to have ill-treated hostages in Beirut while acting for Hizbollah. Evidence is sketchy apart from a racy journalistic account[21]. Of other armed opposition movements — Renamo and SWAPO in southern Africa, the opposition groups of Central America, *Sendero Luminoso* in Peru, and so on — little is known to us. On occasions some have taken captives and sometimes they exerted stern discipline on suspected informers within their own movements[22]. Any doctor working within that environment could easily be pressured to assist in harsh treatment.

Assessing the evidence

Our consideration of the evidence for medical involvement in torture is broken down into the following: examinations prior to torture; presence, examination or treatment during torture; medical examination or treatment after torture; false certification after torture. Some prisoners, of course, have the misfortune to meet hostile or unhelpful medical personnel at several points throughout their stay in detention.

Examination prior to torture

The role of the doctor in examining prisoners entering a place of detention is potentially a protective factor in the prisoner's interests. Indeed, Amnesty International called for such examinations as one of its "12 Point Program for the Prevention of Torture" which was published in 1984[23] and incorporated in the BMA *Torture Report* of 1986. The same provision has been adopted in international human rights instruments. For example, the Body of Principles for the Protection of

---

21 Thomas G. *Journey Into Madness: Medical Torture and the Mind Controllers*. London: Bantam, 1988.

22 According to the 1990 *Amnesty International Report* (p.173) "SWAPO representatives acknowledge that prisoners [held in camps in Angola] had been tortured". SWAPO won power in Namibia at the UN-supervised election in 1990, committed to introduce human rights reforms after 60 years of rule by South Africa. In the case of Renamo, this organization has carried out brutal attacks on health clinics, schools and other institutions in Mozambique (see chapter 8) though the role of medical personnel in its activities is not known to us.

23 Amnesty International. *Torture in the Eighties*. London: AI Publications, 1984.

All Persons under Any Form of Detention or Imprisonment (1988) specifies at principle 24 that:

> A proper medical examination shall be offered to a detained or imprisoned person as promptly as possible after his admission to the place of detention or imprisonment, and thereafter medical care and treatment shall be provided whenever necessary....

However, as Phillips and Dawson have noted, there appears to be:

> a clear distinction to be drawn between the doctor acting on behalf of the prisoner and at his request, and acting on behalf of the adminstration. In the former role, a doctor is acting entirely properly in attending to need and alleviating distress; in the latter, however, he is not only part of the process that is causing the distress but by virtue of his professional standing he is lending that process some spurious respectability since he appears to condone it.... The problem is that in practice it is extremely difficult to separate the two. Examining a prisoner before he is tortured is more straight forward, since the only reason for such an examination is to pronounce the prisoner fit to undergo duress and therefore must be wrong. But examining the prisoner afterwards provokes the dilemma, since it could be in the prisoner's interest or in the interest of the torturers.... In practice, however, it is extremely unlikely that any doctor allowed to examine a prisoner in such circumstances would be a free agent, and that his treatment and opinion would not be used by the torturers.[24]

Indeed, there is much evidence to suggest that doctors or other medical staff who examine prisoners do not always act with the necessary clinical independence and in fact sometimes actively collaborate with security or police in the torture of prisoners.

In Chile, during the government of Augusto Pinochet, there was abundant evidence that doctors examined prisoners on entry into the secret detention centres of the *Central Nacional de Informaciones* (CNI, the Chilean security police). The nature of the examination, which appeared to note conditions which could be seriously aggravated by torture, suggested (and subsequent events confirmed) that the main function of the medical examination was to allow for "effective" torture. For example, a man arrested in Arica in the north of Chile in 1983 alleged:

---

24 Phillips M, Dawson J. *Doctors Dilemmas: Medical Ethics and Contemporary Science*. Brighton: Harvester Press, 1985, p.101.

> I was again taken to the first room, undressed and examined by the doctor, who even measured my blood pressure.... Then another interrogation expert, I think, came in and asked, "Have you examined this one yet? Is he good for a going over? The answer was affirmative.[25]

The same pattern occurred in other Chilean cities:

> A male detainee arrested [in Valparaiso in October 1983] alleged that he had been asked by "someone who appeared to be a doctor" about previous illnesses, about the symptoms and about the medication he was taking. After examining him with a stethoscope and asking him if he suffered from asthma, he called out that [the detainee] could take it."[26]

An investigation into medical involvement in torture in Chile carried out by the Colegio Médico de Chile found that the role of the doctor in the work of the security police was highly developed. According to a report published by the Colegio Médico in 1986:

> One physician who had worked for the security forces told us that there was an entire clinical structure in place with specialists, resources, shifts, joint consulting, and even 'emergency calls' to respond to any imprudence or ever-zealous action by other officials that put the life of a detainee in danger. It should be understood that these 'emergency services' are provided to those patients who, because of their deteriorated physical or mental state, are often unable to request their own medical attention.
>   As our investigations continued, we discovered that physicians working within this system had medically examined detainees before torture and then issued certificates of good health after torture.[27]

Unfortunately, the return to democracy in Chile has not put an end to allegations of torture and of medical involvement. In September 1991, Amnesty International reported that more than 30 complaints of torture had been submitted to Chilean courts since the coming to power of the Aylwin government in March 1990.

One man complained that after his arrest he had been beaten, subjected to *teléfono*, deprived of food, and subjected to mock execution. According to his statement he was examined by someone

---

25 Amnesty International. *Human rights in Chile: the role of the medical profession.* AI Index: AMR 22/36/86, September 1986.

26 *Ibid.* p.2. Similar allegations were published in: Amnesty International. *Recent torture testimonies implicating doctors in abuses of medical ethics in Chile.* AI Index: AMR 22/29/84, May 1984.

27 *The Participation of Physicians in Torture.* A report of the Chilean Medical Association, 1986. *Op. cit.* p.68.

carrying out medical duties, after which torture continued[28]. The detaining authority, the *Carabineros*, denied this and other torture allegations, stating that "all of the detainees mentioned [by the Chilean parliamentary human rights commission] were examined by medical professionals, both when they arrived and when they left the police stations without any visible or evident sign of injuries consistent with torture...".[29]

Presence, examination or treatment during torture

The most charitable interpretation one can put on the presence of medical personnel during the interrogation of a prisoner is that they are there to ensure the interrogation doesn't go "too far". Such a role was proposed by the Parker Committee's report on events in Northern Ireland in 1972 which suggested that:

> a doctor with some psychiatric training should be present at all times in the interrogation centre, and should be in a position to observe the course of oral interrogation.[30]

This role was opposed by the BMA and was rejected by the British Government which accepted a minority report of Lord Gardiner[31] which held such a role of the medical profession to be unacceptable. Since that time, the two main international ethical codes relating to prisoners — the Declaration of Tokyo of the WMA and the Principles of Medical Ethics of the UN — have both specifically proscribed a medical presence at any procedure where cruel, inhuman or degrading treatment might be inflicted. Moreover, presence during torture would be contrary to human rights law.

The overwhelming body of evidence of medical participation in torture indicates that the role of the doctor is not to guarantee a humanitarian presence to help save the prisoner from the excessive enthusiasm of dedicated interrogators; rather the doctor is there to support the torturers. In some cases the testimony given by prisoners

---

28 Amnesty International. *Chile: Reports of Torture Since March 1990*. AI Index: AMR 22/03/91, September 1991, p.15.

29 *Ibid.*, p.6. The case cited here was not one of the five cases referred to by the Human Rights Commission.

30 *Report of the Committee of Privy Counsellors appointed to consider authorised procedures for the interrogation of persons suspected of terrorism. Op. cit.* p.9 (para.41).

31 *Ibid.* [Minority Report], pp.11-22.

suggests a reluctance on the part of the doctor to play the role assigned to him or perhaps an attempt to offer some small assistance to the prisoner. In other cases, the doctor is reported to play a consistent and malevolent role.

Continuing allegations of torture in Chile include isolated reports of apparent medical involvement. A man arrested by the *Carabineros* in Santiago on 9 August 1990 alleged that he was given electric shocks to the genitals, chest and feet, and subjected to *submarino*, as well as other forms of torture. He alleged that, while under torture, he was examined by a woman performing medical duties, following which torture continued[32].

Two doctors cited in an Amnesty International report on El Salvador spoke to a detainee in May 1990 as if he were about to experience a necessary but unpleasant medical treatment. The report quoted the detainee as saying that:

> "...two other persons entered the room and introduced themselves as doctors. They examined me, and checked me all over. One of them said to me that 'you must put up with it.... There is nothing we can do.' I was cold and I was coughing. They said 'you must get through this'. Then they both left."
> After this his interrogators began to give him electric shock torture.

Another case mentioned in this report cites a doctor as reassuring a prisoner he had nothing seriously wrong following beating — "that he was just suffering from the results of the blows he had received". A follow-up report on human rights abuses in El Salvador recorded the allegation of a detainee that he was continually interrogated, had his testicles trodden on by a woman and was then examined by someone he took to be a doctor who gave him some pills.[33]

Turkey has a well-documented record of systematic torture, particularly since the military coup of September 1980. The role of doctors in this torture varies from that of intervention to protect prisoners through to assistance to the torturers or neglect of prisoners who are taken ill. For example, Gazi Eke was arrested in Elbistan in the mountainous region of south-east Turkey on 9 January 1989. At the trial of Mr Eke and 19 other defendants on 13 March 1989, he was not able

---

32 Amnesty International. *Chile: Reports of Torture Since March 1990, op. cit.* p.16

33 Amnesty International. *El Salvador: Killings, Torture and Disappearances.* AI Index: AMR 29/27/90, 24 October 1990, p.12. *El Salvador: Amnesty International's Continuing Concerns.* AI Index: AMR 29/02/91, March 1991.

to give coherent testimony and said that he had been beaten on the head and had suffered from epilepsy. His lawyer asked that he be medically examined to establish his state of mental health. Amnesty International quoted his testimony, given shortly after the hearing:

> On 10 January [1989] we were brought to Kahramanmaras Police Headquarters. On the same day we were taken to the Emergency Ward of Kahramanmaras State Hospital. I told the doctor that I was suffering from epilepsy and that a German doctor had predicted bad consequences if I received beatings and blows, in particular on my head. The doctor, however, told the police that I was in good health.... [Later] I was tortured several times with breaks of some hours in between. After that I completely lost any sense of time....[34]

Another defendant in the same hearing, Oguz Yaman, alleged that he had to be taken to Mersin State Hospital after losing consciousness during torture at Mersin Police Headquarters. He testified in court that:

> I was detained on 18 January 1989. On 19 January I was taken to Kahramanmaras Police Headquarters. On 20 January I had to be taken to Kahramanmaras State Hospital and was forcibly fed [Oguz Yaman had gone on hunger strike in protest against the ill-treatment]. On 21 January I was taken to Mersin State Hospital and again given serum. Next to Mersin Police Headquarters there is a health centre. The doctor there supervised the torture and advised the police officers how long torture should be applied.
> At Mersin Police Headquarters I was stripped naked, my legs and arms were tied to the ground and I was given electric shocks to my penis and other parts of my body. The doctor then ordered the officers to stop this torture and I was hosed with ice-cold water. At the end of the day I was left in a draught of cold air to dry....[35]

Petersen[36] describes incidents of torture occurring in Venezuela in 1989, including several alleged incidents of medical assistance in that torture. For example, one 32-year-old man was arrested on 4 March 1989 and taken to the headquarters of the *Dirección de Inteligencia Militar* (DIM) in the capital Caracas. There he was immediately threatened and subjected to attempted strangulation.

---

34 Amnesty International. *Turkey: torture and unfair trial of political prisoners. Case studies between August 1988 and August 1989.* AI Index: EUR 44/101/89, October 1989, pp.8-9.

35 *Ibid.*, pp.9-10.

36 Petersen HD. Torture in a democratic country, 1989. *Danish Medical Bulletin*, 1990; **37**:556-9.

This provoked one of his attacks of rapid heart rate and difficulty in breathing .... He was examined by a man whom he took to be a doctor. The pulse and blood pressure were measured, and he was allowed a little rest.

There followed during the next 24 hours a period of frequent interrogation and torture.

On most occasions when systematic torture was used against him, the doctor was present, instructing the torturers, e.g. application of electric shocks was not allowed .... On one occasion ... he was again examined medically [and] his blood pressure was found to be high; consequently he was given some tablets.

A recent account of a trial of prison personnel in Yugoslavia on charges of ill-treatment of prisoners throws light on the role of the prison doctor in the abuses. The trial, which took place in Leskovac in Serbia from December 1989 to March 1990, sought to establish the guilt or innocence of nine prison officers and two administrators who were charged with criminal abuse in the form of systematic beatings of 41 ethnic Albanian prisoners. They were arrested on 28 March 1989 during a period of demonstrations against the introduction of legislation withdrawing the 'autonomous' status of the predominantly Albanian province of Kosovo. Detailed and consistent allegations were made by former detainees that on entry into Leskovac prison they were physically and verbally abused.

Some detainees testified that the beating began as soon as they crossed...into the room where the doctor sat. Others were not beaten until after their interview with the doctor.
  [One prisoner] stated that he was clubbed as soon as he entered the doctor's room, and then, "the doctor did not examine me, only asked whether I had any chronic diseases.... Guards clubbed me (again) until I fell...."[37]

Although the prison doctor was not on trial he was required to give evidence. He stated that:

he neither saw nor heard any violence or signs of mistreatment toward the detainees while they were at Leskovac. The presiding judge confronted Dr Rasic with his previous testimony in which he denied being present in the admission rooms, and claimed to have heard cries, blows and screams

---

37 Physicians for Human Rights, Johannes Wier Foundation. *Yugoslavia. Mistreatment of Ethnic Albanians: a Case Study*. The Hague: Johannes Wier Foundation, 1991, p.9.

of agony from an adjacent office. Dr Rasic could not explain the inconsistencies in his testimony. He stated that his present testimony was correct and that his previous statement must have been misunderstood.

Dr Rasic was then confronted with [a] former detainee..., who explicitly claimed that Dr Rasic was present while he was beaten.[38]

Other testimony by ex-detainees presented serious evidence of complicity in the ill-treatment.

The former detainees consistently testified that the doctor was present during the admission procedure, interviewed them only superficially about chronic diseases, did not physically examine them, and was intermittently present while they were beaten. They further testified that no doctor examined them upon their departure from Leskovac prison. Several detainees testified that Dr Rasic instructed the guards to proceed with the beatings, and some gave detailed accounts of the doctor's role.[39]

In summary, the court heard *prima facie* evidence of possible breaches of medical ethics and Yugoslav law by the prison doctor. The fact that this did not lead to any charges being laid against him could be interpreted as suggesting that the prison doctor was not seen as having an obligation to protect prisoners. The response of the Yugoslav and Serbian Medical Associations to this case is not known.

Medical examination or treatment of prisoners after torture

After a session of severe torture, the prisoner may require immediate medical attention to save his or her life. Evidence made available to the Working Party made clear that doctors assisting victims of torture after they have been removed from the torture chamber acted with a variety of motives. The obligation to provide treatment when requested or in case of emergency applies equally in the case of the torture victim. However, three ethical factors come into play in such a situation — at least in principle. The first is that the doctor is enjoined by the Declaration of Tokyo not to condone or tolerate the torture and is thus obliged to note the torture and report it. Secondly, the doctor must pay due attention to the consent of the prisoner to any treatment the doctor proposes. This may require the doctor to be sensitive to a desire by the prisoner to refuse treatment because of the unbearable suffering he or she is being subjected to (though of course it may be impossible for the

---

38 *Op. cit.* p.12.
39 *Ibid.* p.12.

prisoner to express any coherent view in the circumstances). Thirdly, the doctor must assess the best interests of the prisoner and recommend measures which coincide with those best interests. The return of the prisoner to a prison cell and to the control of military personnel clearly is not in the prisoner's best interests though the doctor may be in a very weak position to influence the decision concerning the prisoner's fate. The extent to which the doctor can be expected (or empowered) to play an ethical protective role will be discussed in chapter 9.

While many prisoners are given medical treatment after torture, doctors who play a vigorous denunciatory role appear to be in a minority. On the contrary, some appear to go out of their way to condone torture. In one case a doctor interviewed on British television seemed prepared to justify the torture of Palestinian prisoners and, by prohibiting access to the alleged victims in his hospital, effectively suppressed information. In early 1991, the BBC television journalist, Charles Wheeler, filmed an exchange with Dr Ali, Director of Farwania Hospital in Kuwait, following the country's liberation from Iraqi occupation.

When permission was sought to interview Palestinian patients in a closed ward, Dr Ali denied their existence but later added on film: "If we tortured them, it is because they deserved it".[40] While the remark was made following a conflict situation in which serious atrocities had been committed by Iraqi invaders, such an attitude is not acceptable from health personnel. In other conflict zones, there appears to be evidence still emerging to demonstrate medical impartiality despite atrocities committed by participants; an example is the current Serbia/Croatian conflict. This, and the invasion of Kuwait, and their impact on medical personnel are discussed in chapter 8.

As far as we have been able to judge, the evidence from torture victims who have subsequently spoken of the medical treatment they received is mixed. With the notable exceptions of the relative minority of cases where a specific complaint has been brought against an individual doctor, most victims did not single out the doctor for condemnation as on the side of the police or security agents. Nevertheless, the significance that can be attached to such omissions, given the victim's vulnerable state, is unclear. It seems highly probable that, in most cases, the doctor who sees the torture-injured prisoner

---

40 BBC Television: *Newsnight*; 18 March 1991.

plays a role which is seen by the prisoner as helpful or, at worst, cautious[41].

The evidence relating to medical care given after the fact of torture was, by the nature of our enquiry, focused on the unethical. The main form of abuse brought to the attention of the Working Party related to refusal to treat, or to inadequate or negligent treatment.

In December 1987 in Mauritania, protests against the execution of three black military officers alleged to have been involved in a coup attempt were followed by the arrest of several members of the black community in the capital Nouakchott. One of them later described the torture inflicted upon him in a police station located in the front of the Mauritania Red Crescent offices in Nouakchott:

> For three days, I was subjected to [torture].... They tried to make a hole in the tendon at the back of my knee with a piece of iron, in order to insert an electrode. When they didn't succeed they tried with a piece of bone. A few days later, they tied a weight to my scrotum with string and my testicles swelled. Then they put hot pepper in my eyes and broke five of my teeth. When my mouth became infected I was brought to the hospital. The Algerian doctor there refused to give medical attention, saying that I was dying. I could not either stand up or walk and was kept for 31 days before being transferred to a civil prison.[42]

In southeastern Turkey, where there has been a continuing conflict between the army and the illegal Kurdish Workers' Party (PKK), there are persistent reports of the torture of alleged members and sympathizers of the PKK. Amnesty International reported allegations that three trade unionists charged with support of the PKK "were beaten, hosed with ice-cold pressurized water and given electric shocks during interrogation".

> One of the former detainees also alleged that they had not been properly examined by an official doctor. He said that they had been taken to the doctor blindfold and, in the presence of the police who had threatened to take them back for interrogation, had been asked whether they bore any

---

41 It is possible that a prisoner has relatively low expectations of what a doctor can provide and it is for this reason that prisoners do not see cold or unhelpful treatment as particularly reprehensible. The study of Allodi and Cowgill cited below [note 65] refers to the "neutral" attitude of doctors who, by any account, failed to treat their torture victim-patients with the attention they deserved.

42 Amnesty International. *Mauritania 1986-1989: Background to a crisis. Three years of political imprisonment, torture and unfair trials.* AI Index: AFR 38/13/89, November 1989.

wounds or marks of blows. For fear of being tortured again they had replied negatively and the medical reports therefore contained no reference to marks of blows.[43]

Two cases of individuals from the Middle East were related to the Working Party by the Medical Foundation for the Care of Victims of Torture, where both were interviewed within the past year. The first, a young man, was detained for an extended period by security agents. He was subjected to beating over the head and body, was suspended with his arms behind his back and was given electric shocks to various parts of his body and cigarette burns to his hands. He was held blindfold during torture. He was kept in harsh conditions and not permitted visitors. He attempted a hunger strike but was forcibly fed. At three points during his detention he saw doctors. The first time he was seen by a doctor through the bars of his cell. The doctor did not examine him but apparently recommended that he be hospitalised. After six weeks detention and after a particularly savage episode of torture he was taken to a hospital where he was examined and given an injection; a few hours later he was returned to prison. The third time he again was taken to a hospital, interviewed by a doctor and then returned to the prison.

The second case was that of a woman who was arrested and held for several months in solitary confinement. She was tortured during interrogation by beatings to the feet and whipping, sleep deprivation, burning and being forced to adopt uncomfortable postures. She suffered a miscarriage which she attributes to her torture. Some hours after the miscarriage she was taken to a place where she was examined under anaesthetic by a doctor. She was then returned to her cell without any medication and torture was then resumed[44].

In the Philippines, where during the Marcos period there was "little direct evidence that military or police medical personnel *systematically* transgressed their ethical responsibilities by participating in torture" there were cases where detainees alleged that they were treated with "indifference or outright hostility"[45]. After the arrest of a psychology

---

43 Amnesty International. *Turkey: torture and unfair trial of political prisoners. Case studies between August 1988 and August 1989.* AI Index: EUR 44/101/89, October 1989.

44 Identifying details have been omitted from these accounts to protect the individuals concerned.

45 Claude RP, Stover E, Lopez JP. *Health Professionals and Human Rights in the Philippines.* Washington DC: AAAS, 1987, p.28.

student in 1983 an intelligence officer repeatedly punched him in the stomach and neck, the beatings only stopping when his mother arrived. When he was examined three days later, the doctor signed a medical certificate stating that he had no signs of ill-treatment despite his complaint and evident bruising.

There appears to be a significant problem with regard to the adequate documentation of torture-related sequelae. While some doctors are prepared to state unambiguously that torture occurred[46], the Working Party received evidence that some doctors failed to carry out examinations with due care or, in regrettably too many cases, appeared to falsify medical evidence. For example, in Chile, the medical association reported that it was:

> aware of numerous cases in which physicians have examined victims of torture shortly before their release and failed to report the existence of torture-related lesions....Their examining physician issues a health certificate stating that everything is normal. The physicians' signature is almost always illegible. In addition, the physician fails to note his identification number on the certificate.[47]

On the other hand apparently neutral forensic evidence which fails to state the likely cause of lesions noted or of death can provide evidence to those who can interpret it. For example, a medical certificate written by a doctor examining a woman alleging rape in police custody in India, noted that she had sustained a torn fourchette and, despite the absence of any comment on the probable cause of such a significant injury, it clearly supported the woman's story of sexual assault.

In some cases, the evaluation of evidence of torture is the subject of significant differences of opinion between examining doctors. For example, a 40-year-old Indian Sikh with Canadian citizenship was arrested in Amritsar, Punjab, on 2 November 1987 while visiting India to see a relative. He was later tortured by members of the Central Reserve Police Force. According to his petition to the Indian Supreme Court he suffered electric shocks "first to the penis, then in the anus, thereafter under the armpits, temple of the head and ultimately the

---

46 Rarely with the clarity of the Medical Superintendent of Arawa General Hospital, Bougainville, Papua New Guinea, who concluded a post-mortem report thus: "Sir it is my opinion that this person was tortured to death and then shot". Amnesty International. *Papua New Guinea: human rights violations on Bougainville, 1989-1990*. AI Index: ASA 34/05/90, 1990.

47 *The Participation of Physicians in Torture*. A report of the Chilean Medical Association, 1986, *op. cit.* p.73.

nose". He also alleged that he was beaten and had his legs pushed apart to 180 degrees[48]. Two weeks after his arrest, he was medically examined by Dr Anand Gopal Singh Bawa of the Civil Surgeon Office in Amritsar.

> His report recorded two bruises on the body of Balkar Singh, one of 5cm by 4cm on the sole of his right foot and another of 5cm by 3cm on the back of his right forearm. He stated that Balkar Singh complained of pain in his inner thighs and in the left side of his chest. Dr Anand Gopal Singh Bawa found that the injuries had occurred between 11 and 16 November and that they were caused by a blunt instrument.[49]

Balkar Singh was transferred to the Central Jail, Amritsar, where a second medical examination was carried out on 25 November 1987 by the prison doctor, who reported no sign of external injury. He did not exclude the possibility of ill-treatment but noted that Balkar Singh had not complained of torture. The Indian Government refused a medical examination by an outside expert and later reported to the United Nations Special Rapporteur on Torture that:

> [when] Balkar Singh appeared before a team of Canadians who had been granted consular access to him [he] deliberately pretended to limp and levelled allegations of torture and illegal confinement. However, Mr Singh could not show any visible mark of physical injury and the allegations of torture were not substantiated.[50]

After his release in October 1988 he was examined by a team of doctors in Canada who concluded that his complaints, certain signs including increased pigmentation on the sole of the right foot, and a psychiatric evaluation of post-traumatic stress disorder were all compatible with his story of torture. Legal investigations into the allegation of torture have been hampered by failure of police to cooperate with the investigation and the lack of an independent expert medical examination of the prisoner in the period shortly after the alleged torture.

Pressure to assist in human rights violations

Doctors can be placed under considerable pressure to assist the authorities, particularly in the cover up of torture, deaths in custody or

---

48 Amnesty International. *India - Human rights violations in Punjab: use and abuse of the law.* AI Index: 20/11/91, 10 May 1991.

49 *Ibid.* p.25.

50 UN document E/CN.4/1990/17, p.25; cited in *ibid.* p.26.

other abuses. For example, following the death under torture of a 40-year-old man in Delhi, the Resident Doctors' Association of the All-India Institute of Medical Sciences claimed that the South Delhi police chief, "in connivance with a senior doctor, had been trying to pressure Dr R.K. Sharma to change the [post-mortem] report and give TB as the cause of death"[51]. The post-mortem carried out by Dr Sharma was reported to have shown that the deceased had been assaulted and that a head injury was the cause of death. A magisterial enquiry implicated three policeman and one assistant public prosecutor in the killing and charges were laid against the accused[52].

In South Africa, a direct challenge to the role of the doctor in protecting his patients occurred in 1986 following a township demonstration where the crowd was fired on by the police. The police subsequently requested patients' files from the Alexandra Clinic. The Clinic's director, Dr Tim Wilson, refused on the grounds of medical confidentiality. The files were forcibly seized by police and eventually returned when Dr Wilson complained that patient care was being obstructed by the lack of files. The then Director-General of the Department of National Health later observed that the Alexandra Clinic "was the only clinic ... which had refused to cooperate with police"[53].

A similar event arose in 1988 when Dr Paul Davis was subpoenaed to divulge the names and addresses of patients of his who were included in a study of the effects of detention published in 1985. The reason given by the government for this order was that it was necessary to identify those in the study in order to investigate their allegations. For Dr Davis the central problem was clear[54]:

> The issue of confidentiality has to be addressed. In South Africa, there is no such thing as doctor-patient privilege in a court of law. One has to make the conscious decision to uphold the principle of confidentiality in spite of the possible demands and probable punishment by courts.
>
> It is as sobering as it is frightening to confront the notion that institutions that purport to dispense justice force one to break one's word to one's patient. ...

---

51 Police action sparks ire of doctors. *Indian Express*, 1 October 1986.

52 Information from Amnesty International.

53 van Es A, van Gurp M. *Health Professionals and Human Rights in South Africa*. The Hague: Johannes Wier Foundation, 1987, p.52.

54 Davis P. Medical responses to the problem of torture in South Africa. In: Gruschow J, Hannibal K [eds]. *Health Services for the Treatment of Torture and Trauma Survivors*. Washington DC: AAAS, 1990, p.118.

> The central issue is that the patients have not given their permission for me to reveal their names.

The court dismissed the case against Dr Davis in February 1989 when it was revealed that he no longer held the medical records being sought.

A similar confrontation occurred in Chile in the late 1980s when the authorities tried to seize all the medical records held by the human rights organization, the *Vicaria de la Solidaridad*, supposedly in the course of an investigation of an Arms Control case which involved a Vicaria doctor, Ramiro Olivares, and others. It was widely seen in Chile as an attack on the Vicaria and was condemned internationally. The Vicaria successfully resisted the police attempts to gain access to the records. This case is discussed in more detail in chapter 8.

Which doctors torture?

Most doctors in Britain, indeed throughout large parts of the world, do not work with prisoners at risk of torture. Prisoners are kept apart from the rest of the population and usually are served by a special prison medical service. Countries which provide medical services to prisoners solely through the normal civil health service, such as Norway, appear to be the exception. This may change. In England and Scotland, there were government moves in 1991 to encourage general practitioners to undertake prison medical service. These were generally opposed by the BMA, which supported calls by prison reformers for specialised training for doctors undertaking such work. In May 1991, a private member's bill to abolish the Prison Medical Service was introduced into the House of Commons but with no chance of adoption[55]. Nevertheless moves for reforming the PMS in the direction of greater involvement of outside doctors appear to be on the agenda[56].

However, in most countries, it is those doctors working in prisons and other places of detention, police surgeons, who assist in forensic aspects of police work and military doctors, who may be required to work with detained soldiers and prisoners of war, who are most likely to confront the issue of ill-treatment and torture. Where doctors in such institutions are isolated, or have worked for many years in the same

55 Smith R. Further call to abolish the prison medical service. *British Medical Journal*, 1991; 302:1359.

56 Directorate of Prison Medical Services (Home Office). *Contracting for Prison Health Services: A Consultation Paper*, August 1991.

institution, or work under the overriding responsibility of the prison authorities, there is a risk of their independence, and capacity to assert their ethical principles, being diminished. If the doctor is "one of the boys" — a functionary dependent on officer colleagues for friendship or good will, or to civil superiors for professional advancement — then there is a basis for exerting considerable pressure on them not to be obstructive, or possibly to actively assist the torture to go "smoothly".

In addition, these are precisely the doctors who are most likely to be required to observe some form of "contract of obedience". A doctor faced with a choice between a moral oath and a military oath may find the conflict extremely difficult to resolve. One step to resolving this potential conflict suggested by the Uruguayan medical association is to confer civilian status on doctors working within the armed forces — i.e. civilian status with regard to their medical duties. In the UK, doctors in the armed forces finding themselves in conflict with their superiors over a medical ethical issue can appeal to the BMA for guidance and support. We discuss this further in chapter 11.

If police, prison and military doctors are most likely to be the personnel seeing tortured prisoners, they are not the only ones. During widespread military operations, it is possible for local doctors to be asked to provide medical services, including to prisoners. Equally, doctors working in hospital casualty departments or intensive care units may also find themselves dealing with serious trauma inflicted on a prisoner. In a notorious Chilean case, a seriously ill prisoner, Federico Alvarez Santibañez, was transferred from the custody of the security police to the Penitentiary Hospital where a medical student recorded:

> multiple contusions on the cranium, thorax and extremities. Pallid, rapid and shallow breathing, pain in sternum, multiple thoracic pains, nausea, heavy perspiration, labored breathing. Lucid and oriented. Extensive bruising around the eye sockets.[57]

His condition worsened and he was transferred to another specialist hospital where he died. The day of his transfer from security police custody:

> he was "examined" by Dr Luis Losada Fuenzalida in his capacity as a CNI [security police] physician. It is obvious that Dr Losada placed the interest of the CNI before ... his patient's because the health certificate he signed reads as follows: "The undersigned physician has professionally

---

57 *The Participation of Physicians in Torture.* A report of the Chilean Medical Association, 1986, *op. cit.* p.73.

examined Federico Renato Alvarez Santibañez, C.I. 646.500-8 of Santiago, and found him in good health and showing no wounds of any kind. Santiago, 20 May 1979." In May 1986, the Chilean Medical Association expelled Dr Losada.[58]

In some cases of prisoners admitted to hospitals, the police accompanying the prisoner insist on certain actions which can impede the treatment which doctors want to administer. For example, in Turkey prisoners have been chained to their hospital beds. In July 1987, the Turkish journal *Yeni Gündem* reported that prisoners in Samsun State Hospital were chained to their beds and that all prisoners in Ankara's Numune Hospital had been chained to their beds some years earlier[59]. In a case where a prisoner was taken to Tepecik Chest Hospital for treatment for tuberculosis in 1986, the supervising military commander ordered that he be chained to his hospital bed.

> When the doctor demanded that the patient be untied for treatment the guards refused to remove the chains, citing their orders. [The prisoner] remained chained to his bed until his discharge from hospital [12 weeks later].[60]

In the Israeli Occupied Territories also, a detained Palestinian woman was reported to have been bound to a bed during the final stages of her pregnancy, her feet being free during the birth itself. A 29-year-old man was also reported to have been bound to his bed during his period in hospital. Other cases were also alleged to have happened. The Israel Medical Association was reported to have promised to check these reports and to make an official protest[61].

In countries of refuge such as Britain, doctors may well encounter victims of torture in the form of refugees or asylum seekers. While this is a separate issue, it does raise questions about the sensitivity needed to avoid inflicting further suffering on patients through ignorance. This will be touched on in chapter 7.

---

58 *Ibid.* pp.73-4.

59 Amnesty International. *Turkey: Torture and Medical Neglect of Prisoners*. AI Index: EUR 44/28/88, May 1988, p.9.

60 *Ibid.*

61 The Association of Israel-Palestinian Physicians for Human Rights. *Annual Report 1990*. POB 10235 Tel Aviv 61101, pp.30-1.

Investigating medical involvement

Torture is illegal under international law and frequently prohibited by the laws applying in countries where it is practised. It is not surprising therefore that attempts are made to hide it. In addition, those who have been tortured may not want to report their experiences, either because of the suffering this may cause or because they feel that publicising their story may put others at risk.

We found the extent of medical involvement is similarly difficult to assess. Torture can happen without medical participation, and thus any evaluation of the extent of torture does not necessarily indicate the level of medical involvement unless it is clear that doctors are systematically integrated into the torture process. Few medical associations replied to BMA requests for information on the problem of torture and medical involvement in their own countries[62]. This may be due to the absence of the problem, an absence of evidence available to the medical association or a failure of the association to reply to the BMA request.

An additional difficulty in assessing levels of involvement include the fact that very few convictions or sanctions of any kind have been obtained even in countries where medical involvement in torture is known to have been systematic. For example, in Argentina only one doctor was convicted in a court of law for involvement in torture[63]. In Chile and Uruguay no doctor is known to have been prosecuted for acts of torture or assistance in torture. Finally, there is little detailed published analysis of evidence of medical involvement in the medical literature. While some papers specifically refer to aspects of medical involvement in torture these generally restrict analysis to individual experiences or to sample populations. Allodi and Cowgill, for example, reported that of 41 cases they reviewed, 19 reported that they had encountered 21 doctors during and after their torture:

> In prison four physicians checked the victims and torture continued. Outside the prison twelve doctors maintained a neutral attitude. They did not talk to the patient or inquire about injuries or, if they treated the injuries, they did not offer comfort. Five doctors treated their patients

---

62 The BMA wrote to all national medical associations when the working party was established in 1989. By the end of 1991, only eight bodies had replied and the information gained was limited. In some cases follow-up letters from the BMA were ignored.

63 See chapter 3, note 13, p.25.

ethically, comforting and protecting them. One surgeon refused to allow soldiers to remove his patient from her hospital bed[64].

Rasmussen described the cases of 200 individuals he had examined over a ten-year period. All had been tortured and 41 (20%) reported that medical personnel were involved in their torture[65]. They had been medically examined prior to torture, tortured in the presence of a doctor, had received medical resuscitation during torture or had received non-therapeutic medication. Petersen[66] reported on involvement of medical personnel in Venezuela but the report was an isolated one giving no clue to the scale of medical involvement in torture in Venezuela. In drawing conclusions from these reports, it must be borne in mind that only those who survive their torture and who are willing to testify to their experiences are able to contribute to such studies and, additionally, that countries where doctors were an integral part of the torture process may have been disproportionately represented (particularly Latin America).

Bloche[67] and others[68] have referred to the debate in Uruguay about the collective culpability of all military doctors who practised during the period of military rule. This debate pitted those who believed in individual assessment of charges against those who believed that the military doctor was part of a collective machine for infringing human rights and thus shared a collective guilt. It illuminates the argument over the definition of involvement and guilt and underscores the care with which allegations of guilt must be evaluated. In the event, the procedures adopted by the Uruguayan medical and legal professions to assess charges of collaboration in torture appear to be sophisticated and based on a concept of fair process[69].

The process starts with a *denuncia* (complaint) which must be presented through a lawyer. There follows its presentation to a plenary

---

64 Allodi F, Cowgill G. Ethical and psychiatric aspects of torture: a Canadian study. *Canadian Journal of Psychiatry*, 1982; 27:98-102.

65 Rasmussen OV. Medical Aspects of Torture. *Danish Medical Bulletin*, 1990; 37 (Supplement 1):1-88.

66 Petersen HD, Torture in a democratic country, 1989. *Op. cit.*

67 Bloche GM. *Uruguay's Military Physicians: Cogs in a System of State Terror*. *Op. cit.*

68 Weschler L. *A Miracle, A Universe: Settling Accounts with Torturers*. New York: Pantheon, 1990. Martirena G. *La Tortura y los Médicos*. Montevideo: Ediciones de la Banda Oriental, 1988.

69 Martirena G. *Ibid.* pp.25-6.

session of the National Commission of Medical Ethics where it is either accepted or rejected. If accepted, a team of a doctor and a lawyer from the Commission takes charge of the investigation. The team's findings are presented to the plenary of the Commission which must approve the recommendations by absolute majority. The doctor under investigation is able to contest the finding. The result has been findings of guilt and sanctions against six doctors, a small number given the scale of torture in Uruguay in the period of military rule.

In Chile, the *Colegio Médico* (Medical Association) has pursued a cautious and confidential path towards the investigation and disciplining of doctors found to be involved in torture. Since 1983, the association has undertaken enquiries regarding the alleged participation of 12 doctors. Investigations regarding a 13th doctor opened in March 1991 though, according to Dr Gunter Seelman of the medical association, this last doctor has left Chile apparently to avoid further investigations. To date, six doctors have been penalised, three of whom have been expelled from the College and three temporarily suspended[70]. Again this is a small number considering the long period in which torture was practised with extreme brutality and lack of restraint, and in which doctors appear to have been heavily involved.

Centres working with people who have suffered torture or similar abuses have generally not attempted to assess the extent of medical involvement. However, in a letter to the Working Party, Ms Helen Bamber, Director of the Medical Foundation for the Care of Victims of Torture, drew attention to the significance of the problem of the medical tolerance of torture and ill-treatment:

> Among the people we see there have been a few who report instances of blatant and deliberate abuse by prison, security or military doctors. These examples deserve exposure, investigation, and denunciation. However, we are very concerned that other forms of ethical failure are addressed: the problems of unsympathetic or hostile medical treatment in prisons; lack of medical care (sometimes, it has to be said, due to factors outside the doctor's control); refusal by doctors to document torture; and more generally, the tolerance by medical staff of torture and ill-treatment. These kind of abuses are recounted to us regularly and appear to be widespread. If these basic problems cannot be combated then we should not be surprised if some doctors slide into more active forms of assistance in torture.[71]

---

70 Letter to the Working Party from Mr Patricio Figueroa, Legal Adviser, Colegio Médico de Chile, 8 October 1991.

71 Bamber H. Letter to the BMA, 20 December 1991.

The UN Special Rapporteur on Torture, Professor Peter Kooijmans, made special reference to the involvement of medical professionals in torture in his report of 1990. He renewed his expression of concern in his 1991 report:

> Since the Special Rapporteur continues to receive information that members of the medical profession play a role in the practice of torture, he wishes to reiterate his previous recommendation that professional medical associations take strict measures against such persons who have dishonoured their profession.[72]

Conclusion

The weight of evidence available to the Working Party was such as to allow no other conclusion than that the problem of medical participation, tolerance or cover-up of torture is persistent in some countries and an occasional problem in others. The numbers of doctors involved is impossible to estimate due to the secret and illegal nature of the abuse. In very many cases, there is little evidence that the doctors took any feasible measure to avoid involvement or protect the victim. For such cases, the Working Party has no hesitation in expressing its extreme repugnance of the doctor's behaviour and supporting calls for disciplinary hearings. We believe that the medical profession, and particularly medical associations, must take a more active stand against such unethical and unacceptable behaviour. In doing so, it will need to take into account the need to balance the obligation to report the torture with the need to protect the patient. Clearly, this is an area where medical confidentiality is of the utmost importance.

Nevertheless, the Working Party felt that focusing *only* on the doctors directly involved in gross abuses risks missing the wider perspective both of medical *acquiescence in*, or *tolerance of*, torture (by, for example, professional indifference, fear or lack of knowledge of possible measures).

The Working Party also felt it important to draw attention to medical acceptance or involvement in practices which may fall short of torture

---

72 UN Document E/CN.4/1991/17, 10 January 1991.   Commission on Human Rights. Question of the human rights of all persons subjected to any form of detention or imprisonment: torture and other cruel, inhuman or degrading treatment or punishment. Report of the Special Rapporteur, Mr P Kooijmans, pursuant to Commission on Human Rights resolution 1990/34. See also Professor Kooijmans' 1987 report, (E/CN.4/1987/13, 9 January 1987), particularly pp.9-12: The role of medical personnel in torture.

in the strict sense of the word but which are nevertheless unethical and may be cruel, inhuman or degrading.

While torture and medical involvement in torture will most frequently occur within places of detention or interrogation, knowledge of torture spreads much further. Of equal or greater importance, there is inevitably a wider pattern of abuses than outright torture, particularly in democratic states where checks operate against the worse excesses, and it is important that this phenomenon also be addressed. In some ways medical acquiescence in these types of abuse risks being insidious as it does not provoke the widespread and focused response that reports of medical involvement in torture do.

Although there is currently an abundance of ethical statements and principles available to the profession to address the subject of torture, there is a relative lack of concrete actions which can be brought into play to assist the doctor faced with having to resist pressure to assist in torture. More importantly, there remains the need to develop concrete and feasible measures which states and medical bodies can implement to *prevent* doctors being placed in situations where such choices have to be contemplated. We make recommendations on this in chapter 11.

Chapter 5

Abuse of psychiatry for political purposes

In common with practitioners of other branches of medicine, psychiatrists are not immune to errors of judgment, to breaches of ethics and to lapses in clinical standards which are bound to occur in medicine as in any human endeavour. This chapter does not deal with all such failings or misconduct but with abuses carried out for political reasons or as a result of systematic failures of political will or political control. In this report, abuse of psychiatry refers to abuse of psychiatric procedures, techniques, knowledge and hospitals to detain compulsorily, and "treat", individuals for their political, social or religious views rather than for genuine medical reasons. Whether the detained individuals are or are not genuinely mentally ill is not the determining factor in such detention. What they have in common is that they are not a threat to themselves or to others; rather their views are unsettling to the authorities. The abuse of psychiatric skills in the treatment of prisoners will also be discussed. Other psychiatric issues to be briefly touched on in this chapter include the systematic failure to deliver adequate mental health care in a safe and secure environment. In some examples brought to our attention, the level of care and the conditions within the hospital themselves appeared to be a form of unacceptable ill-treatment.

This chapter will not explore in detail the use of particular psychiatric techniques when used within an accepted psychiatric framework. Our concern about a technique such as electroconvulsive therapy (ECT) is limited to those circumstances where it is used to apparently punitive effect. Other techniques such as aversion therapy, sleep therapy and psychosurgery have not been considered since they appeared to us to be outside the scope of our enquiry. Nor do we enter into the "anti-psychiatry" debate — the argument that there is no such thing as mental illness and that the role of the psychiatrist is solely to be an agent of social control[1]. Discussion of psychiatric aspects of capital punishment will be discussed in the next chapter.

Psychiatry has an in-built capacity for abuse which, according to Bloch and Reddaway, "is greater than in any other field of medicine".

> Why should this be so? Several factors suggest themselves: psychiatry's boundaries are exceedingly blurred and ill-defined; little agreement exists on the criteria for defining mental illness; the mentally ill are often used as scapegoats for society's fears; and the psychiatrist commonly faces a dual loyalty, both to the patient he is treating and to the institutions to which he is responsible.[2]

The diagnosis of mental illness permits the state to detain an individual against their will and then insist on treatment in his or her own interest and in the wider interests of society.

Bukovsky and Gluzman offered this reason for the attraction of psychiatry as a tool for Soviet authorities:

> it enables them to deprive a man of his freedom for an unlimited length of time, keep him in strict isolation, and use psycho-pharmacological means of 're-educating' him; it hinders the campaign for open legal proceedings and for the release of such people, since even the most impartial man will, if he is not personally acquainted with a patient of this sort, always feel a twinge of uncertainty about his mental health; it deprives its victim of what few rights he would enjoy as a prisoner, and it provides an opportunity to discredit the ideas and actions of dissenters and so on.
>
> There is, however, another, no less important side. Dissenters, as a rule, have enough legal grounding so as not to make mistakes during their investigation and trial, but when confronted by a psychiatrist with a directive from above to have them declared non-accountable, they have found themselves absolutely powerless.[3]

In other words, in the monolithic state, psychiatry can be used to bypass normal legal procedures for assessing guilt or innocence and allow

---

1   For a review of the debate see Tantam D. The anti-psychiatry movement. In: Berrios GE, Freeman H (eds). *150 years of British Psychiatry: 1841-1991*. London: Gaskell, 1991, pp.333-47. For a critical updating of "anti-psychiatry" see: Ingleby D. Understanding 'mental illness', in: Ingleby D (ed.) *Critical Psychiatry: The Politics of Mental Health*. Harmondsworth: Penguin, 1981.

2   Bloch S, Reddaway P. *Russia's Political Hospitals*. London: Gollancz, 1977.

3   Bukovsky V, Gluzman S. A Manual on Psychiatry for Dissidents. In: Fireside H. *Soviet Psychoprisons*. New York: Norton, 1979, Appendix 1, pp.92-3.

political imprisonment without the usual odium attaching to such political trials — at least, that appears to be the objective.

Dr Semyon Gluzman, himself imprisoned in a labour camp for ten years for his opposition to psychiatric abuse, told the Working Party that abuses were not the result of "a diagnostic kind of error":

> We know from the history of psychiatry that there's hardly ever any agreement between different schools of psychiatrists. Despite these kinds of differences there's hardly ever a case where practices resulted in somebody who was totally adapted socially and posing no threat to the society would end up confined against their will as a psychiatric patient. I think what happened in my country was a natural consequence of [a] totalitarian regime of thought. And that totalitarianization [affected] not only psychiatrists, but nurses, teachers, doctors.[4]

The Working Party also considers that there are a number of other factors which contributed to the prevalence of psychiatric abuse in the Soviet Union. Among these is the low esteem in which the Soviet medical profession is held. Attitudes which persistently degrade the profession may conceivably work to undermine standards. In addition, the absence of a professional body or a regulatory medical council concerned with medical ethics, and inadequate specialist training, may have contributed to the manipulation of psychiatry for political purposes.

Evidence of psychiatric abuse

In the period from the 1960s up to 1986 (the date of the first BMA report), abuse of psychiatry for political ends was reported to be systematic in the USSR[5], and sporadic in other Eastern European countries such as Yugoslavia, Czechoslovakia, Hungary, and Romania[6]. The difference in the scale of abuse between these countries is striking.

---

4   Dr Semyon Gluzman, testimony to Working Party, June, 1990.

5   See Bloch S, Reddaway P. *Russia's Political Hospitals. Op. cit.*; Amnesty International. *Prisoners of Conscience in the USSR: Their Treatment and Conditions.* [2nd Revised Edition.] London: AI Publications, 1980; Bloch S, Reddaway P. *Soviet Psychiatric Abuse: The Shadow over World Psychiatry.* London: Gollancz, 1984.

6   International Association on the Political Use of Psychiatry. *Information Bulletin.* Published quarterly from 1981. Amnesty International. *Yugoslavia: Prisoners of Conscience.* London: AI, 1982. *Briefing: Romania.* London: AI, 1980. The best estimate of order of magnitude appears to be thousands of victims in the USSR and handfuls of victims in the other countries mentioned.

Why should it be particularly prevalent in the USSR and not elsewhere, even in states based on similar ideologies? According to Bloch and Reddaway, the reasons for this are not clear but they suggest that "the following points may be relevant":

> Communism is a more recent phenomenon in Eastern Europe so there has been less time for the traditional German school of psychiatry to be remoulded to suit Marxist-Leninist ideology. Second, the régimes mostly avoid courting unnecessary unpopularity from their peoples, subtly suggesting to them, indeed, that they would be more liberal if it were not for the military *force majeure* of the USSR — a real threat in view of the invasions of Hungary and Czechoslovakia. Third, because of the overwhelming reality of the *force majeure* there is usually less overt political dissent for the régimes to deal with than is the case in the Soviet Union: dissenters are realistic about their chances.[7]

While these points may indeed be relevant, the reason for the disparity between abuses in the former USSR and elsewhere is a complex one which remains to be fully answered. It appears highly probable that a combination of factors explain its prevalence in states based on bureaucratic communism, the most important of which are:

- an underlying ideology which embodies an unquestioning belief in its unique moral and historical correctness
- a perceived need to have science validate ideology
- a medical profession which takes its ethical starting point and its ultimate obligations from the needs of the state.

In the period prior to the 1983 World Psychiatric Congress, there was concerted pressure on the All Union Scientific Society of Psychiatrists and Narcologists to introduce reforms with the implied threat, and indeed resolutions to the congress, to expel the Society if no changes were introduced. In the event, the Society withdrew from the WPA a few months before the Congress[8]. In 1985, the election of Mikhail Gorbachev as Secretary of the Communist Party of the Soviet Union led at first to hints and promises, and later to concrete examples, of political liberalisation in the USSR. However, change was extremely limited and political prisoners remained in detention including cases in psychiatric

---

7 Bloch S, Reddaway P. *Russia's Political Hospitals*. *Op. cit.* Chapter 1, note 20.
8 Bloch S, Reddaway P. *Soviet Psychiatric Abuse: The Shadow over World Psychiatry*. *Op. cit.*

hospitals. In 1987, the daily newspaper *Isvestia*[9] carried for the first time an article critical of psychiatric practice in the Soviet Union but avoided stating that abuses were systematic and politically motivated. The *Isvestia* article criticised the Civil Commitment Procedure under which individuals could be committed to a hospital in the absence of criminal charges and concluded that the procedure was not only inadequate but widely disregarded in practice. Individuals who were not dangerous had been confined and provisions for a case review of the confinement were widely ignored.

Amnesty International reported that in the period after the publication of the *Isvestia* article, 79 people detained on known or suspected political grounds were discharged from psychiatric hospitals. In an interview published in October 1988 in the weekly *Novoye vremya* (*New Times*), the Chief Psychiatrist of the USSR Ministry of Health, Dr Alexandr Churkin, admitted that two of those discharged had been mis-diagnosed[10]. In early 1989 Amnesty International was told by government officials that since 1987 some 2000 people had been discharged after the USSR Ministry of Health had sent medical commissions to review the cases of psychiatric inmates held for religious offenses, border crossing offenses or expressing anti-Soviet views.

In June 1989, the newspaper *Literaturnaya gazeta* (Literary Gazette) published an article which stated that politics had perverted the psychiatric system in the USSR for decades and said that the leaders of the profession were to blame. This was the first direct critique of the political use of psychiatry to appear in a major Soviet newspaper.

Changes in Soviet law

On 1 March 1988, a decree of the Presidium of the national Supreme Soviet came into force. 'The Conditions and Procedures for Providing Psychiatric Care' replaced a virtually secret Directive of the USSR Ministry of Health — on 'Urgent hospitalisation of the socially dangerous mentally ill' — which had been in force since 1971. The 1971 directive was not a law and therefore was less open to legal challenge and gave no right to appeal. The new statute allowed for legal appeals, and for the appellant to have access to a psychiatrist of their

---

9 Defenceless. *Isvestia*, 11 July 1987. Cited in: *Information Bulletin*. No.15-16. International Association on the Political Use of Psychiatry, July 1987.

10 Amnesty International. *Human rights in a time of change*. AI Index: EUR 46/22/89, October 1989.

own choosing, but was criticised for failing to offer adequate protections to patients' rights[11]. A new draft law was published in July 1990 and revised in October 1990 though the legal framework within the USSR has been overtaken by its demise. However, change is slow and conditions in Soviet mental institutions remain grim. The new regional chief psychiatrist responsible for, amongst others, the high-security hospital of Dvoryanskoye, near Volgograd, was quoted as saying after a visit:

> For a month I couldn't recover from what I had seen.... It was some sort of nightmare! I wouldn't be surprised if in such conditions people lose the habit of human speech and just twitch and completely rot.[12]

Visits of foreign experts, 1989-1991

In February 1989, a delegation of US psychiatrists and other experts visited the USSR at the invitation of the Soviet government[13]. The delegation was able systematically to interview and assess past and present involuntarily-committed psychiatric patients chosen by the visiting team, as well as to discuss treatment methods and procedures with some of the patients, their relatives, friends and, occasionally, their treating psychiatrists. While the delegation initially sought interviews with 48 individuals, it finally saw 15 hospitalized and 12 released patients. (In the two months between the submission of the original list of names to the USSR authorities and the departure from the USSR of the US delegation around half of the hospitalized patients were discharged.) The delegation concluded that nine of the 15 hospitalized patients had disorders which would be recognized in the US as severe psychoses, diagnoses corresponding broadly with those used by the

---

11 Reddaway P. Civil society and Soviet psychiatry. *Problems of Communism*, July-August 1991:41-8.

12 Dr L. Sokolova, cited in: Reddaway, *ibid*.

13 The US delegation was led by a US State Department official, Robert W Farrand; the psychiatric team leader was Loren Roth MD; the scientific director was Darrel Regier MD and the hospital visit team leader was Harold Visotsky MD. The details of the teams methodology, findings and recommendations were given in *Report of the US delegation to assess recent changes in Soviet psychiatry to Assistant Secretary of State for Human Rights and Humanitarian Affairs, US Department of State, July 12, 1989*. It is a little ironic that the US delegation looking into the political use of psychiatry in the USSR should itself be led by a government official and travel under the aegis of the US Department of State. The text of the report is available in: *Schizophrenia Bulletin*, 1989, **15**(4:Supplement):1-219.

Soviet psychiatrists. One of the hospitalized patients had been diagnosed as schizophrenic though the US delegation saw no evidence of mental disorder. Among the 12 released patients examined, the US team found that nine had no evidence of any past or current mental disorder; the remaining three had relatively mild symptoms "that would not typically warrant involuntary hospitalization in Western countries. All these patients had medical record diagnoses of schizophrenia or psychopathology".

> The broad Soviet concept of mental disorder diagnoses in general, and schizophrenia in particular, was apparent in the medical record diagnoses of schizophrenia or other psychotic disorders in 24 of the 27 patients interviewed. This high number of schizophrenia diagnoses exemplified the problem of 'hyperdiagnosis', as verified by a finding of only nine closely matching current diagnoses by both the Soviet and the US interviewing psychiatrists.[14]

Commenting on the US report, two staff members of the USSR Academy of Sciences, Drs Borodin and Polubinskaya, accepted some criticisms and rejected others.

> The Soviet side accepts the critical comments regarding the use of sulfazin and of atropine comas. At the present time, the USSR Ministry of Public Health has developed guidelines for a ban on using these medicaments in psychiatry. ...
>
> While agreeing that individual instances of the use of medicinal preparations for the purpose of punishment took place in the past, we cannot agree with the American specialists' conclusion concerning the continuation of such a practice into the present time. If people in the past reacted to such instances indulgently, now the issues of using medicinal preparations only for medical purposes are strictly monitored.[15]

The commentary continued that:

> In the medical practice of the USSR in general, and not only in psychiatry, it is not the accepted custom to discuss with patients the methods for treating them, except for cases where a physician is the patient.[16]

---

14 *Ibid.* p.29.

15 Preliminary Soviet Response to *Report of the US Delegation...*, *12 July 1989*, ibid. pp.5-6.

16 *Ibid.*

In the months preceding the Eighth World Psychiatric Assembly in Athens, there was considerable debate about the possible re-entry of the All-Union Society into the WPA[17]. In the event, in October 1989 the Society was conditionally readmitted on the basis of having made a public acknowledgement of the existence of previous psychiatric abuse and having given an undertaking to review any existing or further cases and to introduce and support reforms to the psychiatric system and new mental health legislation. It was also agreed that the WPA should send an international commission within one year to review the situation and, if political abuse was found to be continuing, a special session of the General Assembly (of the WPA) could be convened to consider the suspension of the All-Union Society.

From 22 to 25 October 1990 a three member team of the WPA — Dr Jim Birley (UK), Prof. Parameshvara Deva (Malaysia) and Prof. Loren Roth (USA) — were in Moscow to negotiate a WPA visit with officers of the All-Union Society. Detailed arrangements were agreed, with it being envisaged that ten to 15 mutually-agreed and consenting patients would be interviewed in depth. The visit was arranged for March 1991 though the All-Union Society postponed the visit due to lack of hard currency to pay for the WPA team's accommodation. The WPA team subsequently spent three weeks in the USSR in June 1991.

Despite the agreements which had been reached between the WPA and the All-Union Society regarding cases to be reviewed jointly by foreign and Soviet psychiatrists and the importance of including the treating doctors from the Soviet side, things did not go smoothly. The delegation concluded that:

> the All-Union Society did not cooperate with the planning and in the prosecution of this part of the Visit [basic organization of interviews and interviewing teams] in a way which we had a right to expect of professional colleagues in the WPA. There was virtually no attention to detail, nor to ensuring that effective arrangements were in place. In some

---

17 There was intense debate and lobbying on the issue of the readmission. The Royal College of Psychiatrists and the Royal Australian and New Zealand College of Psychiatrists and the American Psychiatric Association urged that the All-Union Society not be readmitted until it had made the clearest steps to reverse its then current practices and organized the release of all victims of psychiatric abuse. The Secretary-General and President of the WPA felt that the Soviet Society had done enough to permit readmission. See the account of the readmission debate in *IAPUP Bulletin*, Number 23, January 1990. For a review of the period between the two congresses see Reddaway P. The WPA and Soviet psychiatry, 1983-1989. In: van Voren R (ed.) *Soviet Psychiatric Abuse in the Gorbachev Era*. Amsterdam: IAPUP, 1989.

instances, in ensuring that the treating psychiatrists were available for the interviews, the Protocol had been totally disregarded.[18]

A list of 15 possible cases for examination and evaluation was sent to the All-Union Society in January 1991; a further nine cases in February and a final case a few weeks later. Of these, 15 were selected for examination during the visit but for various reasons ten cases were seen by the WPA delegation. All ten had been diagnosed by Soviet psychiatrists as suffering from schizophrenia. Seven of the ten cases had been seen by Special Commissions since March 1990 and diagnosis had been revised in three cases, there was dispute with the Commission in two further cases and confirmation of diagnosis in the remaining two cases. By contrast, the WPA team, after reviewing case notes and the results of their own interviews, confirmed the diagnosis of schizophrenia in only one case and noted:

> It is clear, from this small and highly selected group, that there is still a wide gap between Soviet criteria for the diagnosis of schizophrenia, and the criteria used internationally in other countries. Equally important, it indicates that the diagnosis is still over-used in the Soviet Union *even when judged by Soviet diagnostic criteria.*[19] [emphasis in original]

The team found that there was a complete failure to address the issue of rehabilitating the victims of earlier abuses and a mechanism to achieve this was not in place. However, no new cases of political use of psychiatry were uncovered and the WPA decided in November 1991 not to convene an extraordinary General Assembly of the Association to discuss the subject. The position of the All-Union Society will therefore be discussed at the Ninth Assembly in 1993.

The rehabilitation process

Since the 1960s, Soviet human rights activists have maintained a protest about the political abuse of psychiatry. The earliest campaign within the Soviet Union itself to secure the release of a victim of psychiatric abuse concerned the mathematician Alexander Volpin. Volpin was interned in psychiatric hospitals on five occasions, the last time being in February 1968. But some of those who had campaigned for Volpin soon ran into

---

18 *Report by the World Psychiatric Association Team of the Visit to the Soviet Union (9-29 June 1991).* Royal College of Psychiatrists, London, July 1991, p.9.

19 *Ibid.* p.11

difficulties themselves with the authorities. One of these was General Piotr Grigorenko who already had been interned in a Special Psychiatric Hospital for one year and would be re-interned in 1969 for political reasons. In time, the case of Grigorenko was to be considered a test-case, by which later attempts at reform might be measured.

In 1971, Dr Semyon Gluzman wrote a psychiatric report on General Grigorenko. Gluzman came to the conclusion that Grigorenko was mentally healthy and had been committed to psychiatric hospitals for political reasons. The result of this declaration was a sentence of seven years' labour camp and three years' exile in Siberia for Gluzman and continued psychiatric detention for Grigorenko.

Almost exactly 20 years later, in October 1991, the official "diagnosis" on General Grigorenko, who had been twice incarcerated for his defence of human rights, was formally reversed. His case was re-examined over a six-month period by a special commission of psychiatrists, headed by Professor Modest Kabanov, Director of the Psychoneurological Institute in St Petersburg (Leningrad). The conclusion of the commission was that the general had been of sound mind when admitted to hospital in 1964-65 and from 1969 to 1974 for championing causes such as that of the Crimean Tatars[20]. It remains to be seen whether the thousands of lesser known victims of psychiatric abuse will receive due acknowledgement of their suffering and proper compensation. The cases of both Grigorenko and Gluzman are further discussed in chapter 8.

Other recent reports of psychiatric abuse

Romania

In Romania, there have been allegations of some individual cases of psychiatric abuse for more than a decade[21]. In addition to individual cases, there is evidence that psychiatric hospitals were used as short-term detention centres[22]. For example, prior to the 1982 Inter-University Sports "Olympiad", more than 600 dissidents were detained

---

20 Rich V. Soviet Union: Grigorenko "of sound mind". *Lancet*, 1991; **338**:1197-8.

21 See Amnesty International. *Romania Briefing*. London: AI Publications, 1980; *Information Bulletin No.6,* International Association on the Political Use of Psychiatry, March 1983.

22 Johannes Wier Foundation. Report on prison health care and psychiatry in Romania. In press.

and kept out of public view in psychiatric hospitals. Those doctors protesting against this abuse were disciplined.

After the fall of President Ceausescu, further allegations of abuses were made though it has proved difficult to confirm these. One family, whose members were alleged to have been victims of confinement for political reasons and whose cases featured in British press stories[23], was examined by a commission including independent psychiatrists which found their psychiatric diagnosis and treatment justifiable on medical grounds[24]. A presentation of evidence by Romanian psychiatrists at the House of Commons on 7 November 1991 confirmed that it is difficult to arrive at a clear picture of the present situation. Those giving testimony were not agreed on whether there had been new cases of psychiatric abuse since the fall of Ceausescu. They nevertheless testified to the existence of a deliberate policy of psychiatric abuse during the Ceausescu years and the briefing document prepared for the session named three prominent psychiatrists alleged to have been involved[25]. The possibility was also raised that sane individuals who had been interned for political reasons subsequently become mentally ill due to the conditions to which they had been subjected. It is difficult to confirm this. What is clear, however, is that psychiatry *was* abused for political reasons and that, as in the CIS, the rehabilitation and compensation process has not really begun. More generally there remain major difficulties in improving the mental health care system in Romania. The possibility that further cases of psychiatric abuse in that country will come to light in the future cannot be excluded.

Cuba

Although Cuba has been politically linked to the USSR since the US severed relations with Cuba shortly after President Fidel Castro came to power in 1959, few significant allegations concerning the political abuse of psychiatry in that country appeared before the late 1980s.

---

23 The case of the family received publicity in European newspapers as an example of Romanian psychiatric abuse. See: *European*, 9 December 1990. Torment of Romania's rebels: Hundreds remain locked in asylums. *Times*, 16 January 1991, p.17.

24 Comments made by representative of Romanian Embassy, London, at a Parliamentary briefing at the House of Commons. See note below.

25 *Romania's Psychiatric Prison Hospitals: Report prepared for Parliamentary Briefing Session*, 7 November 1991, House of Commons; Jubilee Campaign-Parliamentary Human Rights Group. A Jubilee Campaign press release, 7 November 1991, names five psychiatrists.

Amnesty International and Americas Watch both published reports referring to cases of possible unwarranted hospitalization and ill-treatment of political prisoners[26]. These reports referred to the major psychiatric hospital in Havana and the Gustavo Machin hospital in Santiago de Cuba in the southeast of the country. In 1991, a report on alleged abuse of psychiatry in Cuba was published in the USA[27] which presented cases of ill-treatment in psychiatric hospitals going back to the 1970s. As Vladimir Bukovsky notes in an introduction to the report, the evidence contained in the report suggests that neither the theories of the Serbsky school of forensic psychiatry nor the legal procedures in place in the former USSR are used in Cuba — i.e. prisoners are not diverted from the court system to special psychiatric hospitals as a substitute for political trials in the normal court system.

> There is no political need for sophisticated diagnostics, no sudden epidemic of "sluggish schizophrenia" among dissidents, no Cuban equivalents of Dr Lunts or Professor Morozov [Soviet psychiatric theoreticians at the heart of political psychiatry]. Quite a few dissidents were diagnosed as sane, or not diagnosed at all, before being sent to the psychiatric gulag and subjected to electric shocks....
>
> In short, this is not yet a political use of psychiatry as we know it but rather a bad imitation of it....[28]

However, it presents serious allegations that prisoners end up in the forensic ward of psychiatric hospitals in Havana and Santiago de Cuba where they are subjected to ill-treatment including electroconvulsive therapy without anaesthesia or muscle relaxants. The reported use of ECT in the forensic wards appears, at least in many of the cases cited, not to be an appropriate clinical treatment for the diagnosed state of the prisoner — in some cases the prisoners appear not to have been diagnosed at all. Conditions in the forensic wards have been described in appalling terms and apparently are in stark contrast to the other parts of the psychiatric hospitals which are said to be modern and well-kept.

In August 1981, the Marxist historian Ariel Hidalgo was arrested and charged with "incitement against the social order, international solidarity and the Socialist State" and sentenced to eight years'

---

26 Amnesty International. *Cuba: the human rights situation*. AMR 25/07/90, December 1990; *Human rights in Cuba: the need to sustain the pressure*. Washington: Americas Watch, January 1989.

27 Brown CJ, Lago AM. *The Politics of Psychiatry in Revolutionary Cuba*. Washington: Freedom House, 1991, 217pp.

28 Bukovsky V. Preface. In: Brown CJ, Lago AM. *Ibid*. p.xii.

imprisonment. In September 1981 he was transferred from State Security Headquarters to the Carbó-Serviá (forensic) ward of Havana Psychiatric Hospital where he remained for several weeks:

> Once inside, I realised I was at the complete mercy of a hundred men — convicts from different prisons, the overwhelming majority of whom were violently insane.... The doctors never crossed the shadows of the bars and the orderlies only entered when they had to remove someone forcibly to be subjected to electroshock treatment.... The most repulsive acts imaginable took place there, including rapes and beatings of defenceless elderly persons.[29]

While the thrust of the report focuses on abuses attributed to junior staff (and in particular one frequently-named nurse), the general conditions alleged could not exist without the knowledge or encouragement of senior professional staff. No independent monitoring agency is known to have visited the forensic wards of Cuban psychiatric hospitals. Amnesty International reported its impression that the Havana Psychiatric Hospital appeared to be clean and modern but was not permitted to investigate one of the forensic wards and the existence of the other was denied by the hospital authorities interviewed[30].

The issue of human rights abuses in Cuba remains a captive of the Cold War, with a barrage of anti-Cuban rhetoric and economic sanctions emanating from the US. There remains a need for more independent and impartial investigation of human rights in Cuba. The Cuban government could signal its goodwill by opening up the forensic psychiatric wards for impartial and expert inspection.

Germany

Following the March elections in 1990, the then East German parliament established a committee to investigate allegations of psychiatric abuse in Germany. The report of this committee was published in November 1990[31]. As briefly mentioned in chapter 3, the report focuses on the Waldheim Clinic in Hochweitzschen where, it had been alleged, opponents of the government had been detained and treated against their will. The Waldheim clinic was reported to be old

---

29 Brown CJ, Lago AM. *Op. cit.* p.72.

30 Amnesty International. *Cuba: Recent developments affecting the situation of political prisoners and the use of the death penalty.* AI Index: AMR 25/04/88, 1988.

31 See account in *Lancet*, 1990, **336**:1434-5.

and dilapidated and those held there were kept in unsanitary conditions. One example cited in the report was that of a man who, while in an agitated and euphoric mood had wanted to write to President Reagan and to telephone various politicians. He was subsequently taken to the Waldheim clinic where he was detained, in breach of East German law which specified that compulsory detention could only apply where individuals represented a serious threat to others. The picture remains unclear, however, at the time of writing.

Systematic failures in psychiatric practice

In other countries psychiatric practice raises serious questions while not representing the blatant and deliberate political abuses discussed above. These are more in the nature of systematic neglect and failure to introduce reforms and to safeguard detainees' rights. In some countries mental health provision is said to be so bad that mentally ill prisoners are better off remaining in prison than being transferred to a mental institution.

Greece

In Greece, the psychiatric hospitals on Leros and other sites were reported to grossly breach minimal standards for conditions and medical care. Living standards and amenities for staff and inmates were poor and the impression given to outsiders was bleak indeed[32]. Leros represents a failure of political will to address the economic needs of the island's residents as well as a failure of the health infrastructure to deal more adequately with the treatment of the mentally ill, the mentally and physically handicapped and others who have been marginalised in Greek society. The problems faced by medical staff on Leros appear profound and there has been a major problem recruiting psychiatric and other trained staff to work on the island. Recent reports suggest that there is progressive change underway but there is a long way to go[33].

Japan

Long-standing allegations have been made of high levels of involuntary hospitalization of individuals in Japanese mental hospitals. It has been

---

32 Merritt J. Leros: Europe's shame. *Observer*, 10 September 1989; Anon. The lost souls of Leros. *Lancet*, 1989; ii:1112.

33 Grove R. Greece: a Greek tragedy revisited. *Lancet*, 1991; **338**:107-8.

suggested that committal to hospital is used to deal with individuals who cause shame to the family and that hospitalization is frequently a result of social rather than medical factors.

Psychiatric hospitals are mainly in the private sector and the number of in-patients has shown a long upward trend. Hospitalization rates are around 250 per 100,000 population, as many as 95% of whom are compulsorily admitted[34]. (The figure in the UK is around 5%.) Legal protections were minimal — there was no access to a lawyer, no hearing, no notification of reasons for detention or to a legal appeal mechanism and there was widespread international concern about patients' rights in Japan. This led the International Commission of Jurists and the International Council of Health Professionals to undertake a mission in May 1985 to investigate the state of psychiatric practice in Japan.

The report of this investigation[35] concluded that changes recommended two decades earlier had yet to be implemented and urged that such reforms to mental health law be introduced, that there be an improvement and re-orientation of mental health services and that there be improved education and training in the mental health field. The government proposed major reforms in 1987 but these were criticised as inadequate[36].

The International Commission of Jurists, in a 1988 report, again voiced concerns, criticising the conditions provided for patients and pointing to shortcomings of the new legislation. Their preliminary report included 22 recommendations, half of which addressed human rights issues. They nevertheless expressed "a degree of guarded optimism" about the effect of the legislative reforms[37].

A Japanese lawyer active in campaigns for mental health law reform expressed pessimism about the new Act[38], suggesting that attaining full rights for the mentally ill in Japan would be helped immeasurably by the existence of a strong mental health consumer movement and a source of

34 Etsuro Totsuka. Is reform possible? - Japan's Mental Health Act. Paper presented at the Richmond Fellowship International Conference, 20-22 July 1988.

35 International Commission of Jurists. *Human Rights and Mental Patients in Japan*. Geneva: ICJ, undated [1986].

36 Gostin L. Patients or prisoners. *Guardian*, 11 March 1987.

37 International Commission of Jurists' Mission to Japan, April 1988. Preliminary Report and Recommendations. *ICJ Newsletter*. April/June 1988.

38 Etsuro Totsuka. Is reform possible? - Japan's Mental Health Act. *Op. cit.*

community-based mental health care — both, at the present time, distant goals.

United Kingdom

There have not been, to our knowledge, any verifiable allegations of the use of psychiatry to detain people for their political beliefs in the UK. There have been cases, however, where medical evidence of psychiatric illness of prisoners under sentence has been ignored. For example, during the Yorkshire Ripper case, several medical witnesses testified to the prisoner's psychotic state. He subsequently entered the normal prison system rather than be committed to one of the secure psychiatric hospitals[39]. In another case demonstrating the reverse procedure, a man stated by medical witnesses as being harmless was, nevertheless, committed to a mental institution. This may have been the result of the fact that he could not be convicted of any crime despite general press and political concern at his misdemeanour — trespassing in the grounds of Buckingham Palace and entering the Queen's bedroom.

Regular press articles alleging seriously unacceptable standards in psychogeriatric centres, secure hospitals and prisons have appeared in recent years. For example, there have been criticisms of conditions in the Brixton prison medical wing and of the rate of suicides in that prison. Medical staff have to cope with prisoners who should not be in prison. Both HM Inspector of Prisons and the European Committee for the Prevention of Torture and Inhuman or Degrading Treatment or Punishment (CPT) have pointed to the need for major reforms[40].

Of great concern to the Working Party was the apparent erosion of inspection powers in Britain. It was noted that two external inspectorates

---

39 Editorial. Sutcliffe and after. *Lancet*, 1981; i:1241-2.

40 Editorial. A European committee looks at degrading treatment in custody. *Lancet*, 1991; **338**:1559-60. This editorial concludes that the CPT has shown "initiative and imagination" and has given health workers three messages particularly relevant here:
  • objective medical examinations can provide evidence of physical and psychological ill-treatment;
  • the health care of prisoners requires a clearly defined framework independent of the prison administration, providing a quality of care akin to that available in the community;
  • good health care cannot readily be provided in an environment of squalor and unnecessary suffering.
It concludes that the "blame for the piteous state of medical care for prisoners does not lie with those within the prison medical services", and castigates the health establishment for allowing unethical and unsound practices to develop "by neglect".

exist in the sphere of mental health treatment. The Mental Health Act Commission, although limited in the type of case in which it may formally intervene, has access to observe informally general conditions on a wider scale. It thus provides an indirect check to the potential for abuse. In 1969, publicity in Britain about unacceptable standards in psychiatric hospitals caused the government to establish the Health Advisory Service. The powers of the latter appear to have been diminished, however, in that it no longer initiates visits but is dependent upon an invitation by the Health Authority to carry out an inspection.

This limitation in Health Advisory Service powers was thought by the Working Party to be particularly disturbing in the present context of a changing pattern of care in Britain. Although dissatisfaction has often been expressed in the past about the standards in sprawling institutions dating from the Victorian era, the accessibility which they afforded to large numbers of patients by a variety of medical staff, visitors and other outsiders has permitted general conditions to be observed by many people. The present trend is increasingly towards small, more isolated psychiatric units, run by non-medical managers. The transfer of patients into the community, sometimes without adequate support to ensure expert care may, in some ways, present a greater potential for abuse than treating patients on a major site.

The risks to job security in the UK for those who wish to publicise what they see as shortcomings in the health system are not negligible. A nurse and a doctor, whose criticisms of staffing provision within their respective health services were given publicity, were subsequently dismissed and this has led to calls for a charter to protect NHS "whistle-blowers"[41].

Conclusion

The breakup of the USSR and its replacement by the Commonwealth of Independent States, and changes in Eastern European states have led to a marked diminution in the number of new cases of the use of psychiatry to punish or control critics or opponents of government. This is partly a result of slow reforms to psychiatric procedures but also to increasingly rapid political changes which means that behaviour which was deemed criminal and which brought people to the attention of

---

41 Dyer C. NHS whistleblower wants charter. *British Medical Journal*, 1992, **304**:203.

psychiatrists is much less likely to be criminalised and thus the whole question of forensic assessment does not arise.

Equally, the changes, and particularly the new openness, have brought to light a number of new allegations and with time a clearer picture of the nature and scale of such abuses will surface. The recent WPA investigation of psychiatric practice in the then USSR suggested that the capacity for change of the All-Union Society of Psychiatrists and Narcologists and of psychiatric staff in certain hospitals is limited. The All-Union Society however, like the USSR itself, has been overtaken by events and the character of the psychiatric societies which will replace it are, as yet, of unknown character. The diagnostic criteria used in the former USSR are slow to change, however, and while the theories of the Serbsky school remain there exists the possibility of the diagnosis of political views as representing signs of schizophrenia.

While the probability of new cases of abuse appear to be decreasing, there nevertheless remains the crucial issue of the rehabilitation and compensation of those individuals whose lives have been affected by Soviet psychiatric abuse. The WPA saw no evidence to suggest that this is being taken seriously at the time of its 1991 visit and it must remain high on any professional agenda in the new republics.

Scientific pluralism and medical independence in the republics of the CIS remain to be developed. While the state still controls many of the structures and organs of society, some independent associations are organizing themselves. An independent Soviet psychiatric association has been admitted to the WPA — its status has not been clarified at the time of writing — and in Lithuania an independent medical union has been established which is recommending that specialist medical training extend for three years. (At present, medical specialisation means little more that a few months extra study beyond the primary medical degree.)

In countries outside Eastern Europe and the CIS there are issues of concern though they appear to represent inadequate standards, failure of judicial procedures and a lack of effective supervision and review, rather than a government policy which can be traced to the core of political control.

The new principles for the protection of persons with mental illness[42] adopted by the General Assembly of the United Nations in

---

42 United Nations General Assembly Resolution 46/119: Principles for the Protection of Persons with Mental Illness and for the Improvement of Mental Health Care. Adopted by consensus, 17 December 1991.

December 1991 sets out a number of measures which, if acted upon, could improve the protection of the rights of those diagnosed to be mentally ill. However, they require both the goodwill of the mental health professions, and the political will of governments, to be guaranteed.

Chapter 6

Judicial penalties: corporal and capital punishment

> Had I found him faint during the flogging, I would have ordered him taken down.... I beg to say that it is for me a most painful duty to witness such an operation...and I should be most happy to think that I should never again be called upon to witness so disgusting a scene.
>
> Dr James Low Warren, 1846[1]

If torture has a long history, so too do lawfully administered punishments directed against the body. Indeed, in Europe up to the eighteenth century, the two coincided as physical torture was carried out within a judicial and penal framework[2]. However, in contemporary history, corporal and capital punishments are distinguished fundamentally from torture by virtue of the fact that the former are legal and the latter illegal.

Today corporal punishment takes two principal forms: beating — usually by applications of a few or many strokes of a whip, cane or birch, and punitive mutilation — usually amputation of a hand (and sometimes a hand and foot). The former punishments are currently carried out, or provided for in law, in around 20 countries while the latter are restricted to a small number of states basing their jurisprudence on interpretations of religious law.

Capital punishment is provided for by law in more than 100 countries[3], a figure swollen by the recent creation of independent

---

1   Comments made during an inquest into the death of a soldier after flogging, Hounslow, Middlesex, 3 August 1846, cited in Hopkins H. *The Strange Death of Private White*. London: Weidenfeld and Nicolson, 1977, p.169.

2   Peters E. *Torture*. Oxford: Basil Blackwell, 1985; Ruthven M. *Torture: The Grand Conspiracy*. London: Weidenfeld and Nicolson, 1978.

3   Amnesty International. *The death penalty: List of abolitionist and retentionist countries*. AI Index: ACT 50/07/91, 9 October 1991. The figures, accurate to 16 September 1991, were as follows: 44 countries abolitionist for all crimes; 16 abolitionist for ordinary crimes only; 20 abolitionist *de facto*; and 96 retentionist. Changes in Eastern Europe meant that by the end of 1991, *de facto* abolitionist

republics in the former USSR, and is carried out by the following methods: shooting; hanging; decapitation; stoning; electrocution; lethal gas; lethal injection[4]. The first two methods appear to be the most widespread and the last three are used only in the USA. The role of the doctor in the carrying out of the death penalty is not well documented and the clearest evidence of medical assistance at executions is restricted to the USA and one or two other countries. This role will be discussed below.

Corporal punishment

The following account gives a clear picture of one approach to whipping:

> A prisoner who is to undergo corporal punishment is strapped to an apparatus, known as a triangle.... His feet are strapped to the base of the front legs of the triangle. If the cat [a type of whip] is to be administered, his hands are raised above his head and strapped to the upper part of the triangle.... [He] is screened, by canvas sheeting, so that he cannot see the officer who is administering the punishment.... The cat is administered across the [bare] back ... so that the ends of the tails fall on to the right shoulder-blade.
>
> When the cat is to be administered, a leather belt is placed round the prisoner's loins and a leather collar round his neck, so as to protect these parts from any injury that might arise from a mis-directed stroke. Both the Governor and the Medical Officer of the Prison must be present throughout the execution of a sentence of corporal punishment.... The strokes are delivered at deliberate intervals — the normal rate is not faster than ten or fifteen strokes a minute — the time being counted by the Chief Officer of the Prison.
>
> The Medical Officer stands in a position where he can see the prisoner's face, and he has complete discretion to stop the punishment at any time, if he considers that on medical grounds it is undesirable that it should be continued.... At the conclusion of the punishment local dressings are applied, and the Medical Officer gives any other treatment which may be required. In practice, it is only on very rare occasions that the prisoner needs any attention from the Medical Officer....

---

countries increased to 21 and retentionist countries to 106.

4   Amnesty International. *When the State Kills...* London: AIP, 1989. The 1991 *Amnesty International Report* noted that in Iran, one prisoner was executed by being thrown off a precipice. Apparently the law in Iran also provides for crucifixion (as does Sudan) but these forms of execution appear to be very rare.

This account comes from 1938 and describes the practice of whipping as carried out in the United Kingdom up until its final abolition in 1948[5]. The laws relating to corporal punishment in Britain were reviewed by the Cadogan Committee which was appointed in May 1937 and reported in February 1938[6]. The committee recommended abolition of corporal punishment (which was accepted by the government of the day) but the recommendation was not implemented until 1948[7].

There were attempts at various times after 1948 to reintroduce corporal punishment and in 1960 there was sufficient public pressure to induce the Home Secretary, Mr RA Butler, to refer the issue to the Advisory Council on the Treatment of Offenders which reported in November 1960[8].

Despite the conclusion that there was no case for reintroducing corporal punishment, pressure for reintroduction persisted, including from within the BMA. The Annual Representative Meeting of 1961 passed a resolution "That in the opinion of the Meeting, in the absence of proven diminished responsibility, the right to order corporal punishment in certain cases of those found guilty of a crime of violence should be restored to the judiciary"[9]. Over the following year, the matter was considered by the BMA Committee on Medical Science, Education and Research, and the Council, and eventually it was concluded that:

> Further careful study has been made of the report on 'Corporal Punishment' by the Advisory Council on the Treatment of Offenders. The [BMA] Council is satisfied that the Advisory Council has taken exhaustive evidence and that the report contains ample scientific opinion to justify the findings outlined in its conclusions ... that corporal punishment should not be reintroduced as a judicial penalty.[10]

---

5 Report of a Departmental Committee on Corporal Punishment. Cmnd. 5684, London: HMSO, 1938 [reprinted 1952]. Cited in *Corporal Punishment: Report of the Advisory Council on the Treatment of Offenders*. Cmnd. 1213. London: HMSO, November 1960 [reprinted 1961], paragraph 75.

6 Report of a Departmental Committee on Corporal Punishment. *Ibid.*

7 As a judicial penalty, corporal punishment had virtually ceased to be used after reforms in 1861 and, although it was reintroduced for certain crimes in 1863, 1898 and 1912, in practice it was implemented in a very limited way. *Ibid.*

8 *Corporal Punishment: Report of the Advisory Council on the Treatment of Offenders*. Cmnd. 1213. London: HMSO, 1960 [reprinted 1961].

9 Paragraph 272, Supplementary Annual Report of BMA Council, 1961-62.

10 Annual Report of BMA Council, 1962-3, paragraph 155.

National and international laws diverge

For the most part, international human rights instruments have not specifically addressed themselves to the issue of corporal punishment. However, corporal punishment as a disciplinary punishment for prisoners is specifically referred to in the UN Standard Minimum Rules for the Treatment of Prisoners[11]:

> Corporal punishment, punishment by placing in a dark cell, and all cruel, inhuman or degrading punishments shall be completely prohibited as punishments for disciplinary offenses. [Rule 31]

As a result of the Tyrer case in the United Kingdom (Isle of Man) in the 1970s[12], the European Commission on Human Rights and subsequently the European Court of Human Rights ruled that the use of corporal punishment was in breach of article 3 of the European Convention on Human Rights which prohibits cruel, inhuman or degrading punishments, thus effectively ending judicial corporal punishment in Western Europe. This made formal a practice which had been observed in all Western European states. This did not stop a move to reintroduce caning and birching into British law. At Westminster in March 1982, three government backbench MPs attempted to introduce a clause into the Criminal Justice Bill which would have permitted magistrates to order young male offenders aged 10 to 13 to caning, and males aged 14 to 17 to birching[13]. This attempt failed.

While the International Covenant on Civil and Political Rights does not refer specifically to corporal punishment, the Human Rights Committee established under the Covenant to monitor its operation has considered the issue. In "general comment 7 (16)" of 1982[14], it asserted that "in the view of the Committee the prohibition [on torture

---

11 The Rules are included in Annex 3 of Rodley N. *The Treatment of Prisoners Under International Law. Ibid.*

12 Anthony Tyrer was sentenced to three birch strokes to be applied to the bared buttocks in the presence of a doctor on the Isle of Man in 1972. His case is briefly described in: Rodley N. *The Treatment of Prisoners Under International Law.* Oxford: OUP, 1987, pp.249-50. For general discussion of international law and corporal punishment see chapter 10, *passim.*

13 *Guardian* [London], 23 March 1982.

14 See General Comment 7 (16) in United Nations: *Report of the Human Rights Committee,* Official Records of the General Assembly, 37th Session, Supplement No.40 (A/37/40) 1982. *Annex V: General comments under article 40, paragraph 4 of the Covenant.*

or cruel, inhuman or degrading treatment or punishment] must extend to corporal punishment...". Given the expert credentials of this committee some weight must be given to its views.

However, several countries retain corporal punishment within national legislation for use as an alternative, or as an additional, penalty in criminal or political cases[15]. Where whipping is provided as an alternative to imprisonment, the doctor can face an additional dilemma since prisoners may *seek* whipping rather than imprisonment. The doctor's refusal to certify fitness for the punishment may therefore not be welcomed by the prisoner. Even if the prisoner's views are not known to the doctor the dilemma remains since the alternative to the whipping may be a harsh and extended period of imprisonment, separated from their family and perhaps leaving them with no breadwinner[16]. We will touch on this and other dilemmas below.

A number of those countries providing for corporal punishment are present or former Commonwealth countries. For example, Malaysia provides that corporal punishment in the form of up to 24 strokes of the *rotan* (a long cane) can be inflicted as whole or partial punishment for males convicted of drug offenses, rape, kidnapping and firearms offenses. (For youthful offenders, the maximum sentence is 10 strokes.) In addition, whipping can also be imposed under *Syariah* (*Shari'a*) for various offenses under Islamic law[17]. Malaysian law specifies that:

(i) The punishment of whipping shall not be inflicted unless a Medical Officer is present and certifies that the offender is in a fit state of health to undergo such punishment.
(ii) If, during the execution of a sentence of whipping, a Medical Officer certifies that the offender is not in a fit state of health to undergo the remainder of the sentence the whipping shall be finally stopped.

---

15 According to information of Amnesty International and the Johannes Wier Foundation, the following countries permit whipping as a punishment: Botswana, Brunei, Ghana, Iran, Jordan, Malaysia, Pakistan, Saudi Arabia, Singapore, South Africa, Sudan, Swaziland, Tanzania, United Arab Emirates, Yemen; the West Indian states of Antigua and Barbuda, Barbados, Grenada, Guyana, St Lucia, and Trinidad and Tobago; Zimbabwe and Zambia. Australia formally abolished corporal punishment in two of its territories - Christmas and Cocos Islands - in 1991. Zimbabwe changed the constitution and reintroduced whipping after it was declared unconstitutional by Zimbabwean courts. In 1991 the Namibian Supreme Court also ruled that corporal punishment was unconstitutional.

16 Johannes Wier Foundation. *Health Professionals and Corporal Punishment*. The Hague: JWF, 1990, p.6.

17 See Amnesty International. *Whipping: Malaysia*. AI Index: ASA 28/01/90, 24 January 1990.

Singapore sentences prisoners to caning, using a similar procedure to that used in Malaysia[18]. Crimes for which caning is applicable range from rape and "molestation of a housemaid" to overstaying by aliens and "setting fire of national day bunting". Prisoners are certified by a medical practitioner as fit for punishment, strapped to an A-frame with padding over the lower back, and the sentence inflicted in the presence of a doctor. A former Director of Prisons described the procedure in 1974:

> The officer uses the whole of his body weight and not just the strength of his arm. He holds the cane rigidly at arm's length and pivots on his feet to deliver the stroke. The skin at the point of contact is usually split open and after three strokes, the buttocks will be covered with blood.[19]

South Africa also resorts to corporal punishment, with an extraordinary enthusiasm. Parliamentary answers provided by the Justice Minister indicated that between mid-1985 and mid-1990, more than 180,000 sentences of whipping were handed down in South African courts. Of particular significance is the provision in Section 36 of the Prisons Act 8 of 1959 which specifies that:

> Corporal punishment shall not be inflicted before the medical officer has examined the prisoner and has certified that he is in a fit state of health to undergo such punishment ... [and that] the punishment shall be inflicted in private in the presence of a medical officer.[20]

The issue of corporal punishment does not appear to have been widely discussed in penal or medical circles in South Africa though there have been recent signs that the Medical Association of South Africa has changed its view, moving from a position of legalistic acceptance of the punishment to opposition to the medical role in certifying and overseeing the punishment[21].

---

18 The legal provisions are set out in almost exactly the same language as that used in the Malaysian law. See Section 231 of the Criminal Procedure Code of Singapore. The Code states that the number of strokes must be specified at the time of sentence and "in no cases shall the caning awarded in any one trial exceed 24 strokes in the case of an adult".

19 Statement made by Quek Shi Lei, Director of Prisons, Singapore, in 1974. Quoted in *Sunday Times* [Singapore], 13 July 1986.

20 Cited in Amnesty International. *Medical concern: Whippings: South Africa.* AI Index: AFR 53/19/90, 26 March 1990.

21 Information from Amnesty International, June 1991.

Whipping is also a punishment permitted under *Shari'a* (Islamic law). In Iran, Saudi Arabia, the United Arab Emirates, Jordan and countries outside the Middle East such as Pakistan, a variety of crimes are punishable by whipping, usually sexual and property-related crimes.

The Pakistani legislation, which was introduced in 1979[22], sets out very clearly the role of doctors in the supervision of the punishment: "the convict shall be medically examined by the authorised medical officer so as to ensure that ... the punishment will not cause the death of the convict" [para 5(a)]; a sick prisoner will have the punishment postponed until certified fit to undergo it [para.5(c)]; the whipping shall take place in the presence of a doctor in a public place [para.5(f)]; if after the whipping has started, the doctor fears the death of the prisoner, the punishment may be postponed until the doctor certifies fitness for punishment [para.5(m)]. The laws were put into effect under the government of General, later President, Zia ul-Haq. However, after Benazir Bhutto came to power in the elections of 1988, she made a statement during a visit to the USA that there would be no use of corporal punishment under her administration. Despite this, at least two whippings were recorded during the period of her government[23]. As Dr Mahboob Mehdi of the Pakistani organization, Voice Against Torture, has pointed out[24], a change in government does not necessarily mean a change in practices.

[E]ven after the death of President Zia ul-Haq in 1988 and the coming to power of the new government, the process of torture and cruel, inhuman and degrading punishment continues. For example, the public flogging of Fateh Mohammad took place in Haroonabad on 31 January 1989. The flogging was witnessed by thousands of people, including [prison and police staff] and Dr Azhar and Dr Mohammad Bashir, both medical officers. Fateh Mohammad's condition deteriorated after receiving 15 lashes. The remaining 15 lashes were administered after he was revived by the doctors.

In August and September 1990, President Ghulam Ishaq Khan promulgated an ordinance which redefined certain crimes and punishments under the Penal Code of Pakistan. The *Qisas and Diyat*

---

22 The Execution of the Punishment of Whipping Ordinance, 1979. The text is given in full in *Pakistan Times*, 11 February 1979.

23 Amnesty International. *Whipping in Pakistan*. AI Index: ASA 33/11/91, 18 September 1991.

24 Mehdi M. Doctors in Pakistan realise that torture is a 'problem'. *International Newsletter on Treatment and Rehabilitation of Torture Victims*, 1990; 2:6.

Ordinance provides for punishments which are considered cruel, inhuman or degrading by internationally accepted human rights standards. It was promulgated again in January 1991, ordinances lapsing otherwise after 120 days. The *Qisas* (retribution) provisions allow for infliction of injury to the prisoner to an equal degree to that inflicted *by* the prisoner against another party. The injuries (or "hurt" in the terms of the ordinance) for which *qisas* can be exacted include: the dismemberment, amputation or severance of any limb or organ of another person; the destruction or permanent impairment of the functioning, power or capacity of an organ, or the disfigurement of another person; and certain head or facial injuries[25]. The ordinance specifies that *qisas* punishments "shall be executed in public by an authorised medical officer" who is required to have examined the prisoner beforehand and to ensure that the punishment does not cause the death of the prisoner. The actual method to be employed in carrying out the punishment is not specified and presumably left to the doctor to decide.

Also permitted by *Shari'a* as applied in some countries is the punishment of amputation of the left hand (or fingers) and, for repeated crimes, the left hand and right foot — so-called "cross-limb" amputation. Simple amputation is typically provided as a punishment for property-related crimes. The role of doctors in the carrying out, or monitoring, of amputations appears to be important but not essential; it seems that after initial training the punishment is left to prison guards or orderlies to carry out[26]. Medical academics appear to have played a development role in the technology of the punishment. Staff at Tehran University Medical School were reported to have developed a device to amputate fingers or hands[27].

In Sudan, a British-trained surgeon played a central role in the implementation of *Shari'a*-based amputations which were carried out between 1983 and the downfall of the government of President Nimeiri

---

25 Amnesty International. *Pakistan: new forms of cruel and degrading punishments.* AI Index: ASA 33/04/91, March 1991.

26 According to *Arab News*, 22 March 1990, the Islamic Fiqh Academy (a legal body), at a meeting in Jeddah, ruled that doctors should not attempt to reverse a lawful amputation by re-attaching a severed hand but that they could do so if the hand was found to have been amputated in error. This kind of surgery appears to be an unlikely scenario; more typical is the removal of amputees to a hospital after infliction of the punishment where surgeons carry out resectioning.

27 Amnesty International. *Involvement of medical personnel in abuses against detainees and prisoners. Op. cit.* p.14.

in April 1985. Dr Kamal Zaki Mustafa said in a Canadian newspaper interview that he trained guards to carry out the punishment and supervised the "first six or seven just to make sure my system was working all right"[28]. The carrying out of the first two amputations was graphically described in an account from the Sudanese press agency SUNA:

They were seated on each side of an amputation podium, specially prepared, on chairs fixed to the ground with concrete. They had their right hands covered at the wrist with cotton and two prison clinic male nurses tied a band on the convicts' right arms and fixed a string of some medical instrument which is supposed to hold back blood when the hand is amputated. After the male nurses had checked the blood pressure, the convicts had their legs tied with strong leather rope and their eyes (blind) folded.

The convicts ... were talking to the guards and nurses before and after they were seated on the chairs and would from time to time feel their rights hands, which were anaesthetized and dressed with cotton and bands.... At ten o'clock (in the morning) two soldiers of the prison force, dressed in surgical theatre aprons and holding tall sharp sterilized knives, (entered) and each approached his assigned convict. Each convict was held ... by strong prison guards and each amputator, using the sharp end of the knife, simultaneously held the hand to be amputated by the fingers and cut it swiftly and skilfully from the wrist. The cutting operation took about one minute and none of the convicts uttered a word, moved or made a sound.

As they were given local anaesthesia and high doses of sedatives they obviously did not feel any pain, or at least they did not show that they did. The amputators did their job amid cheers of approval from the spectators, towards whom each amputator held the removed part of the hand....

There were stretchers ready...and after the cutting off operation [one prisoner] was carried to one of them, while [the second] walked by himself, guarded, to the other one. They were immediately carried to a waiting ambulance for first aid, and then to the hospital for further treatment....

A doctor who was among the officials attending the amputation operation said each of the convicts was examined by doctors to see how fit they were for the operation, and that the convicts would also be seen immediately by doctors for quick treatment[29].

---

28 *Globe and Mail*, 16 October 1986, cited in: Amnesty International. *Involvement of medical personnel in abuses against detainees and prisoners.*, *Op. cit.* p.14.

29 Sudanese news agency, SUNA, December 1983; see: Amnesty International. *Sudan: amputation and flogging.* AI Index: AFR 54/01/84, April 1984. An *Agence France Presse* account of this event told an essentially similar story adding that "the

Prior to the introduction of the punishment in Sudan a delegation from that country visited Iran to learn the techniques and procedures. After the Nimeiri government fell, the use of amputation as a punishment was suspended.

In June 1989, however, a military coup brought to power a government committed to renewing the application of their understanding of Islamic law. In March 1991, the government announced the promulgation of laws specifying a range of punishments including whipping, amputation, execution by stoning and crucifixion. In September 1991 the first sentences under the new law were given[30].

In August 1991, amputations were reported to have been inflicted in Yemen which, in 1990, incorporated into its constitution a provision that inhumane punishments were prohibited. Doctors are believed not to be involved in the infliction of the punishment.

Nevertheless, in most countries where they are carried out there is a high risk of medical involvement in corporal punishments which by their very nature can cause damage to the body. Indeed, there is an apparent moral dilemma posed by such punishments since, it could be argued, a doctor could lessen the worst effects of such punishment by intervening and stopping the punishment on medical grounds. We will discuss this question below.

As the extracts of whipping laws and regulations cited above indicate, prior to corporal punishment a doctor can be required to evaluate the prisoner's suitability for punishment and to certify his or her fitness for whipping or, alternately, to recommend that they are not fit for the punishment. They may be asked in some countries to confirm the age of the sentenced prisoner. During the whipping the doctor may also intervene to stop its execution though it is not clear on what precise medical grounds such an intervention would be made. How is the doctor supposed to know when to intervene when the flogging itself is clearly injurious to the prisoner and quite serious trauma may be inflicted by the first stroke? How adequately can a doctor be expected to monitor the health of the prisoner without examining him?

---

two who carried out the operation...said that they received four days' training in the surgical theatre of Khartoum Hospital before carrying out their first amputation". AFP, 9 December 1983. Cited in Amnesty International. *Amputations in Sudan.* AI Index: AFR 54/21/83, 20 Dec 1983.

30 Amnesty International. Urgent Action. Amputation sentence. Sudan. AI Index: AFR 54/16/91, 24 September 1991. In 1991 two sentences of amputation of the hand and one of amputation of the hand and foot (so-called 'cross-limb' amputation) were handed down.

Concern about the effect of whipping on the body is not new; it was referred to almost 150 years ago by Dr Thomas Wakley, the West Middlesex Coroner and founder-editor of the *Lancet* who, at the inquest into a British soldier who died after a disciplinary whipping in 1846, asked:

Who knows the force of the shock to the human frame by the system of flogging the skin, which is so fine and sensitive that the smallest prick of a needle may give acute pain?[31]

It is this nonsensical collision between a cruel punishment and the healing nature of medicine which suggests to us that doctors could play a more useful role opposing the use of such punishments (as has the Pakistan Medical Association) than in intervening in individual cases and lending the procedure a medical gloss.

Cultural values and medical involvement

Are criticisms of amputations from those who hold to international codes of ethics a "hysterical reaction of the West" as a Muslim doctor from South Africa wrote in a letter to the *Lancet*[32]? If a society accepts corporal punishments, should not doctors participate in order to minimise suffering? In our own society we can answer this question firmly in the negative but can we answer for others of different cultures? In addressing this question we have to take several factors into account. Firstly, there is an authoritative body of international legal opinion which suggests that corporal punishments fall within the scope of the application of international human rights instruments. Of particular note is the view of the Human Rights Committee which stated in its authoritative "general comment" of July 1982 that corporal punishment should be understood as a cruel, inhuman or degrading punishment[33]. A number of states of different cultures which are signatories of the International Covenant on Civil and Political Rights (ICCPR) nevertheless continue to permit corporal punishment in possible breach of the ICCPR proscription of cruel, inhuman or

---

31 Cited in Hopkins H. *The Strange Death of Private White*. London: Weidenfeld and Nicolson, 1977, p.178.

32 Nadvi S. Amputations and Islam. *Lancet*, 1990, **336**:386.

33 United Nations. *Report of the Human Rights Committee*. Official Records of the General Assembly, 37th Session, Supplement No.40 (A/37/40), 1982. General Comment 7(16), para.2.

degrading treatment or punishment. Where countries are not signatories, they are not formally bound by the terms of the Covenant or its interpretations. However, virtually all states are parties to the Geneva Conventions of August 12, 1949, which prohibit corporal punishment in those situations to which the Conventions apply.

In a wider field, there are a number of guiding principles which also proscribe corporal punishment or, more particularly, medical involvement. For example, the UN Standard Minimum Rules prohibit (at Rule 31) the use of corporal punishment as a disciplinary measure against prisoners, and the UN Principles of Medical Ethics also strictly prohibit medical participation in cruel, inhuman or degrading treatment or punishment. However, as Rodley has pointed out, the UN Principles do not unambiguously preclude medical personnel from evaluating a prisoner as fit for corporal punishment though they can be read as doing so[34]. In this regard the World Medical Association's Declaration of Tokyo is more clearly against such a role and has been interpreted to suggest that corporal punishments are cruel, inhuman or degrading punishments in which doctors should not participate[35].

Another perspective on medical involvement in corporal punishment and international ethical standards is provided by the behaviour of doctors in countries where such punishments either apply or could apply. For example, the introduction of punitive amputations in Mauritania in 1980 met strong objections from the Mauritanian Association of Doctors, Pharmacists and Dentists (AMPHOM) after individual doctors carried out the amputation of the hands of three convicted criminals in the capital Nouakchott in September 1980. After the first amputations, the president of the association wrote to the Minister of Health saying, *inter alia*:

> ...as members of the Mauritanian Association of Doctors, Pharmacists and Dentists, and adhering strictly to the professional codes of medical ethics which prevent us from passing judgment on the principle of carrying out the Shari'a, we ask you as Minister of Public Health to act as our intermediary before the Military Committee of National Safety and before the government, so that steps will be taken to ensure that no doctor takes part in the amputation of hands or in any other act which

---

34 Rodley N. *Treatment of Prisoners Under International Law. Op. cit.* pp.293-6.

35 See: The World Medical Association appeals against torture. *World Medical Journal*, 1981; **28**:22; see also Rodley N. *The Treatment of Prisoners under International Law. Ibid.*

might harm the physical or moral integrity of an individual since our duty is to relieve suffering and to save lives.[36]

In the face of this opposition from the medical profession, two further amputations were carried out in 1982 by medical auxiliaries. *Shari'a*-based punishments ended in Mauritania in 1984 following a change in government.

In Pakistan, there have been no amputations despite laws providing such a punishment having been in place since 1979 and many sentences having been handed down. The reason for the lack of implementation of the sentences is said to be due to the strong opposition of the medical profession in Pakistan and the difficulty the authorities had in finding surgeons to participate[37]. With regard to flogging, it appears that some doctors are willing to play a supervisory role though again there have been protests from Pakistani doctors[38].

In the Amnesty International annual report of 1991, eight countries were recorded as inflicting corporal punishment during 1990; all were either former European colonies or countries implementing a form of *Shari'a*, though these are a minority of states with predominantly Muslim populations. (There are nearly 50 countries which have significant Muslim populations [25% or greater] and 41 which have majority Muslim populations[39].)

A number of African countries — all ex-English colonies — are also believed to practice corporal punishment, sometimes employing foreign doctors (from within Africa) to provide medical supervision[40]. The total number of countries practising corporal punishment, or permitting it by law, is around 20, though documentation of this form of punishment is difficult to obtain.

---

36 Letter from AMPHOM to Mauritanian Minister of Labour, Health and Social Affairs, Nouakchott, 25 November 1980. Copies of the letter were sent to all Mauritanian doctors and circulated abroad.

37 *International Herald Tribune*, 12 February 1979.

38 Pakistan Medical Association (Karachi Branch) adopted a resolution against whipping and medical participation in 1983 and announced it at a press conference. The organization Voice Against Torture has persistently campaigned against the use of the punishment. The Pakistan Medical and Dental Council, on the other hand, has not expressed a view on the medical and ethical implications of whipping. The BMA has not succeeded in getting a statement of principle from the PMDC despite writing several times.

39 Bassiouni MC. *Introduction to Islam*. Chicago: Rand McNally, 1988.

40 Information from Johannes Wier Foundation, Netherlands, January 1992.

To assist Dutch doctors travelling to countries where corporal punishment is carried out, the Dutch government has produced a formal declaration which can be presented to officials in the host country. The declaration sets out the government's view that corporal punishment is in breach of international human rights standards and that:

> The involvement of health personnel in the certification of prisoners or detainees as being fit to undergo corporal punishment should therefore be avoided.[41]

Cultural and religious values and corporal punishments

In addressing the very sensitive issue of cultural values, religious beliefs and their role in prescribing or validating various forms of punishment, it is necessary to commence by noting that the subject to be discussed here is medical involvement in the carrying out of punishments, *whatever the basis on which such punishments are implemented.* However, in order to discuss the role of the doctor in assisting the carrying out of corporal or capital punishment in countries where these practices carry a religious or cultural *imprimatur*, reference to the religious or philosophical basis of the punishment is needed.

Many religions and cultural systems have historically provided for corporal and capital punishments (and indeed for torture). Some might argue that in recent centuries the Anglican Protestant tradition has sought to maintain the use of capital and corporal punishments and there is a need to recognize the role of British colonial policy in the continuing existence of corporal punishment in several ex-colonies.

However, the historic trend has been for the progressive restriction and, in many cases, elimination of such punishments because of their perceived cruelty. There is a view — an erroneous one in our opinion — that Islam is inherently supportive of cruel punishments such as whipping, amputation and execution. There is equally a historic trend in Islam to adjust social conduct in the light of changing social values while retaining fidelity to the five pillars of the Islamic faith. Thus whipping is carried out in no more than one in six of the 50 states with majority Muslim populations. (Around six of the 22 members of the

---

41 Health professionals' ethics and defence of human rights: The Netherlands policy with respect to the involvement of health personnel in corporal punishment. The Hague, October 1988.

Arab League provide for such punishments, making it very much a minority procedure.)

Some commentators have referred to the historical context in which pre-Islamic punishments were ameliorated and controlled through the adoption of Islamic laws and values[42]. In verbal evidence given to the Working Party, Dr Mahboob Mehdi said:

> I think that we should [say] something about Islamic law, because Islam should not be used as a shelter for doing cruel acts. In Pakistan it happened: all those things which were done by [a] dictatorship. Even now the government will say: 'Look, because of Islam we are doing it.' But those are not Islamic things. It is just an interpretation [and] you can use Islam for different purposes.
>
> All the stoning to death, amputation, flogging — all these are pre-Islamic things; they were done before Islam.[43]

The United Nations Special Rapporteur on Torture, Professor Peter Kooijmans, addressed the issue of corporal punishment briefly in his report issued in January 1988. He discussed the relationship between religious values and corporal punishment, noting:

> The fact that highly authoritative religious books recognize or even legalize certain institutions and instruments does not necessarily mean that those institutions and instruments are valid for all places and all times. Slavery may be taken as an example: although slavery was accepted by virtually all traditional religions, it is now generally recognized that it is not compatible with the inherent dignity of man; consequently it is outlawed and seen as one of the most serious violations of human rights. In a similar way, an *opinio iuris* has developed to the effect that the infliction of severe physical or mental pain is irreconcilable with the required respect for man's physical and mental integrity, even in cases where sanctions in themselves are fully appropriate and even called for.[44]

The Working Party felt that focusing only on religious values risked missing the point. There is absolutely no question that the religious

---

42 See comments by Drs Mehdi and Dia, in Amnesty International, Marange V. *Médecins tortionnaires, médecins résistants*, Paris: La Découverte, 1990; (Published in English as *Doctors and Torture: Collaboration or Resistance*. London: Bellew, 1991.

43 Evidence of Dr Mahboob Mehdi, June 1990. At the time Dr Mehdi gave evidence the government of Benazir Bhutto was in power.

44 UN Economic and Social Council. *Report by the Special Rapporteur, Mr P Kooijmans, pursuant to Commission on Human Rights resolution 1987/29.* Document E/CN.4/1988/17, 12 January 1988, paragraph 44.

values of communities and nations ought to be respected. However, criticism of policies practised by states should not be equated with criticisms of religious values. The Working Party attempted to deal strictly with the issue of medical involvement in corporal and capital punishments and did not see that such punishments were inherent to the beliefs of any particular religion. Its focus was on the behaviour of states: it is states which apply laws and states which are bound by international human rights standards. Rejecting medical involvement in corporal punishment reflects the Working Party's view of the doctor as a healer and not as a person who inflicts, or assists those who inflict, punishment.

Capital punishment

The Working Party did not consider the merits of capital punishment as a penalty as this was not within the remit of the ARM resolution. Rather it focused on the role of medical personnel in the preparations for and the carrying out of the penalty and on the ethical dilemmas uniquely posed by this irreversible punishment. Broadly-based consideration of the involvement of doctors in the death penalty was particularly handicapped by the lack of research on capital punishment in general outside the USA and, to a lesser extent, Europe.

As with corporal punishment, the death penalty is a punishment which, by virtue of its effects on the body, has involved doctors in different aspects of the process in many countries. Doctors have historically played a key role in the development or refinement of execution technologies: from the guillotine in the 18th century, through hanging and electrocution in the 1880s to lethal gassing and lethal injection in this century[45]. However, the debate about the role of doctors in executions was never addressed seriously until legislation in 1977 in the states of Oklahoma and Texas introduced execution by lethal injection onto their statutes. This started a vigorous discussion with the weight of argument being against participation[46]. In 1980, the Judicial Affairs Committee of the American Medical Association approved a

---

45 Amnesty International. *Health Professionals and the Death Penalty*. AI Index: ACT 51/03/89, 1989; Jones GRN. Judicial electrocution and the prison doctor. *Lancet*, 1990; **335**:713-4.

46 Curran WJ, Casscells W. The ethics of medical participation in capital punishment by intravenous drug injection. *New England Journal of Medicine*, 1980; **302**:226-30.

statement recalling that the doctor's role was to preserve life where there was a possibility of doing so and that the only possible role for a doctor at an execution was to certify the death of the prisoner. When an execution by lethal injection was scheduled in September 1981, the Secretary-General of the World Medical Association issued a press release reiterating the ethical role of the doctor and concluding that doctors should not participate in an execution though could certify death. This press release was later given formal approval by a resolution of the World Medical Assembly meeting in Lisbon in September 1981 (see Appendices).

Some arguments have been advanced in favour of medical involvement by supporters of capital punishment, usually on the grounds that medical involvement can maximise the good that can come out of the process. For example, Kevorkian has argued that doctors have a positive moral obligation to participate in execution by lethal injection in order to allow the prisoner to donate organs for research or transplantation and thus compensate, in part, for their crime[47]. The philosopher Sheleff has argued that opponents of capital punishment should:

> ... at least accept the execution by lethal injection — so that if all their efforts to save a life fail, they can at least ensure that the act of execution will be a minimum violation of the dignity of the condemned person, and should actively work to make sure that it is so. It is true that by making an execution ostensibly more palatable the abolitionist argument is possibly weakened, but if an execution cannot be avoided, humanistic considerations dictate that the least offensive form of execution be used.[48]

While the latter argument appears not to have found favour within the medical profession, there is certainly a trend in the USA for execution by lethal injection to become a more widely-used technique[49] — probably less for reasons of "humanistic considerations" than those of

---

47 Kevorkian J. Medicine, ethics and execution by lethal injection. *Medicine and Law*, 1985; 4:307-13.

48 Sheleff LS. *Ultimate Penalties: Capital Punishment, Life Imprisonment, Physical Torture.* Columbus: Ohio State University Press, 1987, p.345.

49 In 1977 there were four states with lethal injection legislation (Idaho, New Mexico, Oklahoma and Texas); by 1987, this had increased to 15 states and by 1991, 20 states. Some of these provide for lethal injection as an alternative to other forms of execution. (Information drawn from *Death Row USA*, detailed updated analyses of prisoners under sentence of death in the US published by the NAACP Legal Defense and Educational Fund Inc., 99 Hudson Street, New York.)

cost factors and public acceptability. The technique remains one in which direct medical involvement is a real possibility (see below). In Taiwan and Hong Kong, the possibility of using organs from executed prisoners has moved from a theoretical suggestion to a practical reality. The British Broadcasting Corporation (BBC) reported from Hong Kong in 1990 that surgeons in Hong Kong hospitals were carrying out transplants using organs bought from the People's Republic of China. The organs were believed to have come from executed men[50]. The surgeons involved recognized the moral and ethical arguments which could be made against this process, particularly in the light of possible executions following the Tiananmen Square demonstrations of June 1989, but wished to save lives with the available organs. Further press reports appeared to confirm that the People's Republic of China is involved in the trade of kidneys from executed prisoners to hospitals in the British colony. According to a study by a surgeon from the University of Hong Kong cited by Reuters[51], the fact that prospective recipients could be given appointments for their transplant indicated either that they were scheduled to receive organs from live donors or from executed prisoners. The most common source of organs — victims of accidents — cannot be fitted into a pre-planned time-table. A further report of such transplantations appeared in correspondence columns of the *Lancet* in August 1991. A letter from a Hong Kong doctor stated:

> Kidneys are usually obtained from prisoners who are executed for offenses such as rape, burglary, or political "crimes" against the state. No consent for organ removal is given by either the prisoner or the family.[52]

In Taiwan, some doctors at the National Taiwan hospital urged the Justice Ministry to change the form of execution from shooting through the heart to shooting through the brain in order to allow removal of heart and other organs for research or transplantation purposes. In 1990 the Ministry introduced new procedures for execution[53] and currently prisoners have the "choice" of whether or not to donate organs and thus

---

50 Report on kidney transplants from executed prisoners in China. BBC World Service *News Hour*, July 1990; cited in *Medical Death Penalty Newsletter*, 1991, 3:1-2. Amnesty International, Copenhagen.

51 Study says China transplanted executed prisoners' kidneys. Reuters, 21 June 1991.

52 Siu-Keung Lam. Kidney trading in Hong Kong. *Lancet*, 1991; **338**:453.

53 *China Post* [Taipei], 16 August 1990.

where they will be shot. There was subsequently further speculation in the press about executions and organ donation. The Ministry of Justice was reported to be considering further changes to execution procedures to allow more effective use of organs. Hanging and lethal injections were reportedly being considered and doctors were quoted in the press arguing about the feasibility of killing by lethal injection and later using the organs[54].

The Working Party corresponded with the Heads of Surgery Departments in all of the principal hospitals and in particular with Professor Shu-Hsu Chu of the National Taiwan University Hospital, who defended the practice. Professor Shu-Hsu pointed out that the cultural and religious background of Taiwanese people ordained that bodies should be buried intact if possible, thus making organ donation widely unacceptable. Nevertheless, he considered prisoners would welcome the possibility to atone and donate their organs as "an act of contrition"[55]. A similar purpose for the organ donation was expressed by the Justice Minister, Lu Yu-wen: "The purpose of ... allowing a criminal who is sentenced to death to donate his organs is to help him fulfil the desire of contributing his love to society"[56]. In the first year after the introduction of the law, some 50 executions were carried out and more than 20 prisoners donated organs.

One critic of the practice is Dr Lin Yeon-feong, a member of the Taiwan Association for Human Rights, who has stated:

> I am strongly opposed to this kind of transplantation. In a totalitarian country like Taiwan a judge is not immune to political pressure. Those high up in the system may say that we need more transplant organs, and even those in the medical profession are subject to such political pressure.[57]

It was indeed a concern of the Working Party that prisoners would be pressured to donate organs and that pressure might arise to hand down more death sentences or refuse more appeals in order to treat the thousands of patients awaiting transplantation in Taiwan. It was noted that the new procedure to transplant organs from condemned prisoners

---

54 *China Post*, 25 April 1991.

55 Letter to the Working Party from Professor Shu-Hsu Chu, 2 September 1991.

56 Quoted in: Parry J. Organ donation after execution in Taiwan. *British Medical Journal*, 1991; **303**:1420.

57 *Ibid*.

coincided with a dramatic rise in capital offenses and death sentences as well as very lengthy waiting lists for organs.

Apart from the BMA's opposition to doctors advising on execution methods, it was also concerned that doctors carry out intubation and other preparatory procedures prior to the prisoner's death. The Working Party assumed, but was unable to obtain confirmation from Professor Shu-Hsu, that tissue typing was also performed in advance so that suitable recipients could be prepared to receive the organs as soon as the brain stem death of the prisoner could be established. This suggested the potential for doctors to request certain organs and tissue types to match urgent cases they might have on hand. The Working Party feared that acceptance of the general principles which support this practice would eventually permit executions, and selection of prisoners to be executed, to be scheduled according to surgical requirements.

Even if the potential for abuse were not realised, the Working Party regarded this practice as involving an unacceptable role for a physician. In 1991, the Transplantation Society, an international body of transplantation specialists, decided that use of organs from executed prisoners was unacceptable for reasons similar to those outlined above.

Medical participation in capital punishment

For reasons outlined earlier, discussion of medical involvement in capital punishment in this section is restricted to the practice in the US. Nevertheless, the issues apply in practice or in principle wherever executions are carried out.

The precise criteria by which doctors can be said to have "participated" in an execution remain a subject for clarification. In addition, the ethics of that participation is still under debate. After reviewing the evidence, the Working Party felt it could delineate two broad levels of involvement in capital punishment. When a doctor has acted in a way to assist directly in the carrying out of the execution — by administering a drug, by giving technical advice to the executioner or by monitoring the execution — this clearly is *direct participation*. When a doctor has played an essential role in facilitating the execution — by for example certifying the prisoner fit for execution, treating the prisoner in order to allow execution to proceed, or providing medical evidence contributing to a sentence of death (as opposed to lesser sentences) — then the doctor has *contributed* to the execution. The ethical import of this distinction (if any) will be investigated below. First, however, we elaborate the ways in which doctors can play a role in the death penalty. (Table 1 summarizes the spectrum of medical

Table 1: Possible contact between health personnel and condemned prisoners

Medical contact up to 24 hours *before* execution	<ul><li>No contact [a]</li><li>Examining the prisoner and presenting evidence at his or her trial [b]</li><li>Routine medical care during the pre-execution period</li><li>Attention to psychological or psychosomatic crises</li><li>Evaluation of fitness for execution</li><li>Treating prisoners to make them fit for execution</li></ul>
Contact *during* the last 24 hours [c]	<ul><li>No contact</li><li>Confirming the prisoner's fitness for execution</li><li>Examining the prisoner to find suitable veins for intravenous administration of lethal poison</li><li>Tranquillizing the prisoner</li><li>Witnessing the execution</li><li>Examining the prisoner during the execution to pinpoint the moment of death</li><li>Recommending further application of lethal agents if the prisoner has not died</li><li>Preparing the prisoner for organ donation</li></ul>
After death	<ul><li>No contact</li><li>Examining the corpse and certifying death</li><li>Organ utilisation</li></ul>

[a] In some countries it is apparent that condemned prisoners have little or no access to medical personnel during their imprisonment and doctors appear to play little role during or after the execution.

[b] In the USA it is possible to present psychiatric evidence without having examined the prisoner, basing opinion on hypothetical questions about someone sharing some of the alleged characteristics of the prisoner.

[c] In Iraq there were allegations in the early 1980s that Iraqi doctors had been ex-sanguinating condemned prisoners before execution to provide blood supplies for the war front.

contacts between the condemned prisoner and the doctor; only certain of these contacts are ethically questionable or unethical.)

Contributing to the investigation phase of a capital offense

The physician, and particularly the forensic specialist and forensic psychiatrist, may be required to interview a suspect, or carry out other investigative procedures in order to provide evidence and opinion regarding the cause of the crime under investigation. According to prevailing ethics, such interviews and investigations are ethical provided they are undertaken with the clear consent of the suspect and with a clear explanation of the nature of the interview or procedure. In particular, it is not acceptable for a psychiatrist to interview a prisoner as if he or she were carrying out a clinical interview to assist the prisoner while at the same time attempting to gain information for the purposes of prosecution.

Giving evidence in a capital trial

Medical evidence in court falls into two categories: evidence as to fact and expert opinion. The former is medical information which is *known* by a medical practitioner — for example, that the accused was under treatment for diabetes — and a doctor can be subpoenaed to give evidence of fact in court if the judicial authorities deem it to be relevant to proceedings. The latter — opinion — is an evaluation of medical data given by someone particularly well-qualified to contribute such an evaluation — in other words, an expert. It is with respect to expert opinion that most contention has occurred since some of the reasons for introducing expert opinion are related to establishing whether the defendant is in fact liable to be executed on conviction.

Medical opinion can play an important role in the trial of those accused of capital offenses, particularly in the USA. While there is a long tradition of doctors giving evidence in courts of law, the irreversible nature of the death penalty can literally make the medical evidence adduced in court a matter of life or death and for this reason there has been a lively debate on the ethics of testifying in capital cases. Arguments have been advanced against the presentation of medical evidence, usually psychiatric in nature, in capital trials on ethical grounds because the testimony can have lethal consequences:

> The employment of psychiatrists in trials at law has gone far beyond what society expects from any other type of expert witness. This is manifest primarily in trials where the death penalty is involved. Here we find the

anomaly of a physician, sworn to devote himself to the preservation of human life, dealing out opinions whereby the survival or destruction of another human being hinges on the turn of a word. Many psychiatrists refuse any longer to serve as expert witnesses in capital cases....[58]

Others have drawn attention to inconsistencies and problems with this abstentionist viewpoint. Bonnie, for example, has asserted that placing an ethical prohibition on medical evidence in capital cases would mean that:

> the legal system would be deprived of clinical evidence that is often essential to fair and reliable administration of the law in capital cases. This would be especially problematic in the context of capital defendants or condemned prisoners seeking to utilize such evidence to establish a case for leniency.[59]

He also notes the detrimental implications on the employment situation of the doctor concerned of a voluntary ethical abstention from giving testimony. Bonnie concludes that there is no ethical reason for a forensic evaluator to abstain from professional involvement in a capital case other than where he or she has significant personal prejudices against (or for) the death penalty. He also concludes that a condemned incompetent prisoner who is known to want treatment could be treated ethically but treatment should not be given for the sole reason of preparing the prisoner for execution.

Appelbaum, who has written extensively on the ethical dilemmas and potential ethical infractions of medical involvement in the death penalty[60], has more recently addressed the core issue of medical testimony in capital cases where the testimony can contribute to the death of the defendant. He argues that forensic psychiatry is a distinctly different discipline to clinical psychiatry which is not framed solely within the Hippocratic tradition. He suggests that the obligation of the

---

58 West LJ. Psychiatric reflections on the death penalty. *American Journal of Orthopsychiatry*, 1975, **45**:689-700.

59 Bonnie RJ. Dilemmas in administering the death penalty: conscientious abstention, professional ethics, and the needs of the legal system. *Law and Human Behavior*, 1990; **14**:67-90. [p.68]

60 See for example: Appelbaum PS. Competence to be executed: another conundrum for mental health professionals. *Hospital and Community Psychiatry*, 1986, **37**:682-4; Appelbaum PS. Death, the expert witness, and the dangers of going Barefoot. *Hospital and Community Psychiatry*, 1983, **34**:1003-4; Appelbaum PS. Hypotheticals, psychiatric testimony and the death sentence. *Bulletin of American Academy of Psychiatry and the Law*, 1984, **12**:169-77.

forensic psychiatrist is to the objective truth and cannot be bound by the effects of his findings on the prisoner who is the subject of his evaluations[61]. Clearly we are talking about a very difficult intersection of medicine, with its historic obligation to give primacy to the needs of the patient, and the law, with its impartial disinterest in establishing guilt or innocence and in resolving disputes.

It is not difficult to criticize, indeed demolish, the evidence given by proponents of the death penalty such as Dr James Grigson of Texas. The following extract from a journalist's account of Dr Grigson's testimony in the trial of Aaron Lee Fuller, a 21-year-old white man charged with the robbery and murder of a 68-year-old woman, gives a flavour of the style and content of his evidence. After a 40-minute question by the prosecutor establishing the "hypothetical" profile of a man supposedly sharing the characteristics of the convicted prisoner, the defence attorney objected.

> "The board of trustees of the American Psychiatric Association has reprimanded you for your expression of an opinion as to predictions of future dangerousness have they not?"
>
> Seemingly unperturbed the Doctor replied, "They sent me a letter saying that this will serve as a reprimand."
>
> "And the American Psychiatric Association has labelled your predictions as quackery, haven't they?"
>
> "No, sir, they have not," the Doctor said, still smiling.
>
> "I would object, Your Honour, to any testimony, as not being recognized within the field in which he practises."
>
> "I will overrule the objection," said the judge. And at last prosecutor Smith was able to ask the Doctor for an answer to the killer question.
>
> "Doctor, based upon that hypothetical, those facts that I explained to you, do you have an opinion within reasonable medical probability as to whether the defendant, Aaron Lee Fuller, will commit criminal acts of violence that will constitute a continuing threat to society?"
>
> "Yes, sir, I most certainly do have an opinion with regard to that."
>
> "What is your opinion, please, sir?"
>
> "That absolutely there is no question, no doubt whatsoever, that the individual you described, that has been involved in repeated escalating behaviour of violence, will commit acts of violence in the future, and represents a very serious threat to any society which he finds himself in."
>
> "Do you mean that he will be a threat in any society, even the prison society?"
>
> "Absolutely, yes, sir. He will do the same thing there that he will do outside."

---

61 Appelbaum P. The parable of the forensic psychiatrist: ethics and the problem of doing harm. *International Journal of Law and Psychiatry*, 1990; **13**:249-59.

And that was it. All the 'medical', 'scientific' testimony the jury needed — in any case all they'd get — to justify a judgment that Aaron Lee Fuller was beyond hope of redemption, and ought to be put to death. ... [Later, the jury] took two hours to agree unanimously on a death sentence for 21-year-old Aaron Lee Fuller.[62]

It could be, and has been, argued that the problem with Dr Grigson's testimony is not so much that it is given in an inappropriate forum but that it is scientifically invalid (albeit that it appears to help the prosecution secure death sentences). But what of the forensic psychiatrist (or other medical witness) who attempts to give his or her considered and scientifically reasoned opinion? Equally importantly, what happens when doctors, for reasons of conscientious objection to the death penalty, refuse to testify in capital cases? How can the forensic psychiatrist choose which murder trials at which he or she will present evidence? Is there an ethical argument in favour of one position against the other? We found this a complex and tangled issue where it seemed easier to state what *was* ethical in our view rather than what was not. There seemed to us to be no profound ethical argument against a doctor giving personal evidence or expert opinion in any part of the legal process intended to determine guilt[63]. Provided that a doctor paid due respect to issues such as consent and confidentiality as well as clearly indicating to the accused the nature of any examination, giving evidence intended to elucidate guilt or innocence appears to be a role which is accepted by the judiciary, the public and the medical profession. Our doubts and troubles escalated rapidly when it came to determining, directly or indirectly, whether the prisoner lived or died. While doctors sometimes cannot avoid taking life or death decisions, they usually do so where there are unavoidable pressures influencing them. In the case of capital trials, there is no equivalent imperative. The state may or may not decide to take the life of the convicted prisoner and the doctor is invited to contribute to the process of determining which choice to make. It has been argued that doctors should testify in those parts of the trial where the prisoner's life is at stake, since mitigating evidence may indeed lead to the prisoner being spared execution. This is true of course if the doctor does present mitigating

---

62 Rosenbaum R. On the road with Dr Death. *The Independent Magazine* [London], 8 September 1990, pp.24-32. [quotation from p.28.]

63 We nevertheless accept that some, perhaps many, doctors would feel distinctly uncomfortable being involved in any trial where determination of guilt could lead directly to the death of the convicted.

evidence. But what if the doctor has no mitigating evidence to present? Or if the doctor is retained as an expert witness by the prosecution, presumably because his or her evidence will actively support the prosecution case? Is there an ethical case against such evidence? We believe that presenting evidence on the future dangerousness of a prisoner is fraught with risks and the dangerousness element of death penalty legislation is a poor basis for making life or death decisions. For doctors to make such evaluations without even seeing a prisoner is an unacceptable abuse of psychiatry.

Examining and certifying the prisoner as fit for execution

Clearly certifying the prisoner as fit for execution contributes to the carrying out of the death penalty and this role could usefully be examined in the light of prevailing medical attitudes to fitness assessment examinations and medical approval of corporal punishment. If the latter are unethical, as the BMA believes, then it appears arguable that certifying fitness for the ultimate corporal punishment cannot be less unethical. It is arguably considerably less ethical since there can be no *medical* reason for permitting one execution to proceed and refusing another. Competence for execution is, for some, a strange concept. The Working Party was fortunate to receive evidence from Professor Michael Radelet of the University of Florida. Professor Radelet is strongly opposed to the death penalty personally but believes that it is important that prisoners at least have the chance to benefit from the testimony of concerned and ethical psychiatrists. He suggested that such experts might counter the opinion of the psychiatrists willing to testify consistently that the prisoner is competent for execution even where, in his view, there were grounds for disputing such testimony. The countervailing view, which was raised within the Working Party, was that the long-term objective of consolidating medical ethics should take precedence over short-term interventions in individual cases — that ethical decisions should be made on ethical grounds and not as a result of compromises made with the intention of saving a condemned prisoner's life.

We did not satisfactorily resolve this argument. Nor could we simply resolve the contradiction inherent in the adversarial nature of medical evidence whereby medical evidence introduced to demonstrate incompetence can be countered by state witnesses arguing the contrary. We did note that a doctor testifying on the prisoner's behalf appears to be in quite a different moral position to the doctor testifying for the state. The effect of the latter's evidence of competence is, metaphorically, to provide the state with the syringe filled with lethal chemicals. The execution can go ahead. It appeared to us that the involvement of doctors in contributing to assessments of "fit for execution" will inevitably lead to potential conflicts with basic ethical precepts and these can only be avoided by removing medical personnel from the decision-making process or by ending executions.

Providing medical care in order to ensure that a prisoner is fit for execution

The relationship of the doctor and the condemned prisoner whose incompetence keeps him from the execution chamber is a difficult one. The doctor (or other health worker) faces a very simple dilemma: should I attempt to improve the prisoner's mental well-being and risk the prisoner's life or should I deliberately mismanage the patient in order to ensure his survival? While this may appear to be an extreme hypothetical exercise in medical ethics, in fact it is a real dilemma in the US. Two cases at least have posed the dilemma and have gone to legal adjudication. The first is that of Gary Alvord in the State of Florida. In 1974 he was convicted of strangling three women to death during the course of a burglary the previous year and sentenced to death. His background makes grim reading: he had been first incarcerated at the age of seven and was admitted to a Michigan psychiatric hospital diagnosed a paranoid schizophrenic at the age of 13. He escaped from this hospital and others and carried out further crimes including the 1973 murders for which he was sentenced to death. After a series of appeals he was scheduled to be executed on 29 November 1984. When the issue of his competency to be executed was raised, the Governor appointed a team of three psychiatrists to evaluate Alvord. Their report[64] resulted in a stay of execution of the prisoner and his transfer to a state psychiatric hospital.

The arrival of Alvord at the hospital provoked immediate controversy around the question of treatment objectives[65]. After two years at the

---

64 The report was brief: five sentences stating the psychiatrists' belief that Alvord was incompetent to be executed. "...no details were given as to how the examination was conducted or what medical impairments were found. In short, it was really the psychiatrists, not the governor, who made the decision that Alvord was incompetent." Radelet M, Barnard G. Treating those found incompetent for execution: ethical chaos with only one solution. *Bulletin of the American Academy of Psychiatry and Law*, 1988, **16**:297-308.

65 This is discussed at length in Radelet and Barnard, *ibid*.

hospital, an opinion on his clinical state (but not on his competency) was prepared by a team at the hospital; three outside psychiatrists were appointed by the Governor to conduct a reassessment. In August 1987, Alvord was transferred to Florida State Prison for a competency assessment. However, on the advice of his lawyer he refused to answer any questions. The three interviewing psychiatrists then wrote to the Governor, on prison letterhead, saying that Alvord's refusal to be interviewed showed that he could "respond appropriately" but that they could not "render an opinion within reasonable medical probability as to his competency to be executed". On 15 October 1987, the Governor lifted the stay of execution that had been granted to Alvord in 1984 when he was originally found incompetent for execution.[66]

Restoring an incompetent prisoner to mental health requires the health professional to square the circle: to provide care to the prisoner with the objective of relieving serious medical problems on the basis of trust and confidentiality while at the same time working at the behest of the state which wishes to execute the prisoner. This ambiguity of ends is ethically intolerable and quite a different matter to other situations where a terminally ill patient is nevertheless treated for an acute unrelated illness. The only way to free medical staff from this dilemma is to ensure that those condemned prisoners who are so seriously mentally ill as to fall within the set of exclusions from execution should have their sentences commuted. This of course raises many questions about the pressures on prisoners to "prove" serious mental illness with an accompanying increase in the importance of medical evidence. This risks an increase rather than a decrease in medical involvement in aspects of capital punishment.

A second case with serious implications for mental health personnel is that of Michael Owen Perry whose competence was maintained only by medication with neuroleptics, in this case haloperidol. Perry was sentenced to death in Louisiana in 1985 after the murder of his parents and three other relatives. He had a long history of schizophrenia though he was found competent to stand trial. During his imprisonment he had periodically been placed on anti-psychotic medication. In 1987 the Louisiana Supreme Court upheld his conviction and sentence but ordered the trial court to investigate his competency to be executed. The trial court concluded that he would only remain competent under continuous medication and ordered that he be given such medication — against his will if necessary — so as to render him competent to be

---

66 Radelet and Barnard, *ibid.*, p.304.

executed. The case was appealed to the US Supreme Court which did not decide on the substance of the case but rather referred it back to the Louisiana courts for evaluation in the light of the prevailing standards applying to the rights of prisoners to refuse involuntary medication[67].

While in the end it is the prisoner who should determine whether or not they receive treatment before execution, there are circumstances where the very fact of being on death row can act as a disincentive to the prisoner to agree to medical recommendations. Thorburn[68] recounts the case of a prisoner, Manuel Quintana, who was recommended coronary artery bypass surgery by a cardio-vascular surgeon in March 1983. The prison authorities and doctors were willing to carry out the surgery but the prisoner refused, apparently due to a potentially reversible depression. Given the length of stay on death row in the USA — sometimes more than a decade — as well as the possibility of commutation of the sentence, surgery would have represented a potentially positive step in extending the prisoner's quality and length of life. However, in the absence of treatment he died of ischaemic heart disease in December 1983, four months after the original date scheduled for his execution. Thorburn also raises the role of the doctor in suicide prevention on death row where the beneficent intervention to prevent self-inflicted death is clouded by the fate awaiting the prisoner. While not arguing against prevention of prisoner suicide she does ask whether "[aggressive] intervention [is] merely to serve the state or is it aimed at benefiting the person?"[69]

Advising on, supervising or overseeing the carrying out of the punishment

Doctors have traditionally been involved in contributing to the development of execution technologies and overseeing their use, from the guillotine to the lethal intravenous injection[70]. Over the past two

---

67 New hearing on formed medication of inmate. *New York Times*. 14 November 1990, p.A30. The Supreme Court decision in *Washington v. Harper*, February 1990, established limited constitutional rights for the prisoner to refuse medication. The Harper case is discussed in Appelbaum PS. Washington v. Harper: Prisoners' rights to refuse anti-psychotic medication. *Hospital and Community Psychiatry*, 1990; **41**:731-2.

68 Thorburn KM. Physicians and the death penalty. *Western Journal of Medicine*, 1987; **146**:638-40.

69 *Ibid*.

70 For a summary see Amnesty International. *Health professionals and the death penalty*. AI Index: ACT 51/03/89.

centuries however, there has been a progressive shift in medical ethics towards a strengthening of the obligation on the doctor to avoid any penal function and to maintain a commitment to working for the benefit of the patient. This has culminated in the adoption of international and national standards prohibiting medical participation in executions, in large measure due to the introduction of execution-by-lethal-injection legislation in the USA in 1977. Some legislatures specify by law the exact role of medicine in the process of capital punishment. For example, the state of Oklahoma, one of the first to introduce lethal injection as a method of execution in the USA, framed its legislation in these terms[71]:

> The Chief Medical Officer of the Penitentiary, or the Medical Director of the Department [of Corrections], or a physician designated by the Warden must be present [at the execution; and after the catheter has been inserted] the examining physician shall inspect the catheter and monitoring equipment and determine that the fluid will flow into the vein....The execution shall be by means of a continuous, intravenous administration of a lethal quantity of sodium thiopental combined with either tubo-curarine or succinylcholine chloride or potassium chloride which is an ultrashort-acting barbiturate combination with a chemical paralytic agent. The Department Medical Director shall order a sufficient quantity of the substance....

Several articles in the medical press set out a vigorously stated opposition to doctors' participation in lethal injection[72]. The ethical standards subsequently adopted by the American Medical Association and the World Medical Association permit only the certification of death but no more active role. Unfortunately, these standards are either being consciously breached or are being interpreted in a permissive way by doctors who participate in a direct way in executions. In the state of Illinois, for example, it was reported that in September 1990, three state-licensed physicians helped fit a catheter to the prisoner Charles Walker and inject lethal chemicals into his veins[73]. The reports of medical involvement provoked opposition from doctors in Illinois and

---

71 Oklahoma Department of Corrections. Policy Statement No. OP-090901: Procedures for the execution of inmates sentenced to death. 12 April 1978.

72 See for example: Curran WJ, Casscells W. The ethics of medical participation in capital punishment by intravenous drug injection. *New England Journal of Medicine*, 1980, **302**:226-30.

73 Doctors' role in lethal injection stirs debate. *Chicago Sun Times*. 11 September 1990.

elsewhere. However, attempts to determine the identity of the physicians under Freedom of Information legislation apparently failed.

In the *AMA News* in November 1990[74], information about further executions involving physicians was given, this time taking place in Missouri. Since January 1989, when the first execution in Missouri in 23 years took place, there have been five executions, all by lethal injection. According to the *AMA News* article, in at least two of these cases, physicians have fitted the intravenous lines to deliver the lethal drugs which are dispensed from a purpose-built execution machine. A mixture of sodium pentothal, pancuronium bromide and potassium chloride were the drugs used in Missouri executions. The response of the medical association in Missouri to these reports is not known to us.

The AMA and the Illinois both took steps to strengthen opposition to medical participation. In April 1991, the Illinois State Medical Society resolved to "support amendment of state law to remove any required participation by physicians in the process of executions...". Subsequently, the state legislature took exactly the opposite measures and, in the face of medical opposition, legislated to require the presence of two physicians at an execution and to protect the identity of participants in executions in Illinois. This provoked protests within the medical community[75].

An account of a lethal injection execution in Arkansas in early 1992, which did not go according to plan, provides an awful picture of the process. A 40-year-old man, Rickey Ray Rector, was executed on 26 January 1992 for a murder he carried out in 1981. The execution was schedule to commence at 9pm but it took the execution team 45 minutes to find a vein into which to insert a catheter. According to the administrator of medical and dental services of the Arkansas Department of Corrections, the team expected problems with the execution of Rector who weighed nearly 300 pounds. An Arkansas newspaper quoted him as saying after the execution that:

> We had eight people in there when this all started. The tie-down people were helping, and by the end, we had three more medical people.

The press report continued:

> Byus [the administrator] said the team found a vein within five minutes of entering the room, but the vessel collapsed. "We thought we had it,

---

74 *AMA News*, November 23/30, 1990, p.1.

75 *AMA News*. September 23/30, 1991.

but we didn't," he said. "That's unusual but it happens. He had the spindly veins that collapsed easily. We searched. We were lucky to find a vein at all."...

By the time they found a vein in Rector's right hand, he said, the team already was preparing for a 'cut-down' — a method of cutting into an arm to insert an IV.[76]

Referring to the execution team, Byus said that he didn't "want them categorized as a medical team. That's an ethical question. We weren't there to save a life." Rector was reported to be "aware of the problem" and was praised by Byus: "I'm not going to take anything away from Rickey Ray Rector and the help he gave us with our task....He helped."

Lethal injection is restricted to the USA. However in India, a legal case is being heard wherein a lawyer is petitioning the Indian Supreme Court to permit execution by injection of potassium cyanide solution on the grounds that hanging is cruel. The role of doctors in the proposed scheme was not described[77].

The Working Party felt that existing ethical standards prohibited any kind of involvement in executions and that those doctors acting in the manner reported were infringing well-known international and national ethical codes. One activity, however, which is at a level of involvement less than fully-fledged assistance in the carrying out of the execution and more than merely examining a cold corpse and writing a death certificate, occurs as a result of the presence of a physician at the execution. There have been examples of executions being bungled. It is then for the doctor to declare that the prisoner has not been killed and, effectively giving up responsibility for saving his life, to call for more lethal measures to be applied. In one anecdote reported to the Working Party, a doctor went further than this and allegedly caught hold of a prisoner being hanged and physically assisted the execution which was going awry.[78]

In the USA there have been several bungled executions reported where the doctor's role has been to advise the executioner to proceed with further lethal measures. A recent example of this occurred during the execution of Derick Peterson in Virginia on 23 August 1991. The *Times* reported that "a second jolt of electricity was needed ... when a

---

76 This account comes from the *Arkansas Democrat Gazette*, 26 January 1992.

77 Stay on hearing of execution procedure case. *The Statesman* [New Delhi]. 13 August 1991.

78 Oral evidence to the Working Party from Dr Mahboob Mehdi, June 1990.

doctor found [the prisoner's] heart still beating after the first surge of electricity"[79].

In Taiwan also, during an execution in March 1991, a prisoner remained alive for 34 hours following the first attempt at execution and subsequently was shot for a second time finally causing his death[80]. Surgeons had planned to use his organs for transplantation purposes — an ethical issue which we have previously discussed — but because of delays his organs were not useable. This was at least the second Taiwanese execution in which the first attempt at execution failed to accomplish its objective immediately[81]. In both cases, doctors were required to alert the executioners to the fact that a further attempt to kill the prisoner was required.

Of particular concern in the Taiwanese case is the statement attributed to the Vice Justice Minister that hospitals will be exempted from the normal obligations to attempt resuscitation of an injured person if the person in question was admitted as a result of a failed execution[82].

Regardless of the morality of the death penalty itself, it is contrary to the very heart of medicine for a doctor to assist executioners. As the above examples show, the fact that executions can go wrong places the doctor who is present at an execution in the intolerable position of effectively instructing the executioner whether or not to continue the execution process.

The recent disturbing reports of physician involvement in lethal injection executions in the United States led the American College of Physicians in November 1990 to propose a new standard on doctors and the death penalty and as a result of a resolution it put to the AMA, the latter adopted a resolution itself which included the following points:

> that the [AMA] reaffirm, clarify and publicize its position that it is unethical for physicians, regardless of their personal views on capital punishment, to participate in legally authorised executions, except to determine or certify death...
>
> that the AMA inform state medical licensure boards and certification and recertification agencies that physician participation in supervising or

---

79 Murderer given double dose in electric chair. *Times* [London], 24 August 1991.

80 *China Post*, 17 April 1991, cited in: Amnesty International. *Executions and organ transplantation: Taiwan*. AI Index: ASA 38/11/91, 8 July 1991.

81 *Ibid.*

82 Statement by Vice Justice Minister Lin Hsi-hu, *China Post*, 18 April 1991, cited in Amnesty International, *ibid.*

administering lethal injections is a serious violation of the ethical standards of the medical profession...

that the AMA notify all state medical licensure authorities and, in particular, all physician members of state licensure boards of this position.[83]

The AMA addressed the question again in June 1991 when it adopted a resolution urging state medical societies to reaffirm opposition to physician participation in executions, and to work for a change of legislation in states with criminal codes requiring active physician participation in executions.

Certifying death and signing the death certificate

The problem of distinguishing certification from monitoring and other more active participation is insuperable as long as there is the remotest possibility that the prisoner will not be efficiently killed. The dilemma of what to do when the prisoner is not dead has been discussed above. But what about the propriety of signing a death certificate? Is this, as current ethical standards suggest, a perfectly ethical procedure? Or is it a form of collaboration with the state in the execution process? The Working Party noted the debates which have taken place concerning this issue. A discussion resulting in a declaration against the death penalty by Nordic medical associations appears to have been unanimous in all respects except the issue of certifying death where a majority of associations opposed medical certification of a death from execution while a minority insisted on the legal and moral obligation to certify irrespective of cause of death[84].

The argument against issuing certificates is that it involves possible medical acquiescence in the execution, while the argument in favour is that the doctor's role is to certify "that which he sees" and that unfortunate consequences could be felt by the executed person's family if failure to certify death meant that release of the body for burial or cremation could not occur. The Working Party felt that there would be symbolic importance attached to removing doctors entirely from the execution process by eliminating even the issuing of the death certificate but that it could hardly be deemed unethical for the doctor to determine that death had occurred. Of far more importance, in the view of the

---

83 American Medical Association House of Delegates. Resolution 109: Physician participation in State executions. December 1990.

84 Declaration of the Nordic medical associations, June 1986.

Working Party, is ending the role of the doctor as the one person in the execution chamber who tells the executioner whether or not to continue. In other words, if the doctor is to certify death, then this should be done after an official has confirmed that the prisoner is dead and should take place outside the execution chamber and well after execution has taken place.

Conclusions

The Working Party was presented with clear evidence of medical involvement in the death penalty. This involvement ranged from direct involvement in the carrying out of the execution or advising the executioner as to the need to stop or continue the execution process, through to various forms of medical testimony some of which appears to be given in good faith and others, if not in bad faith, at least in a scientifically unscrupulous and unprofessional way.

Medical participation (and the Working Party believes that participation should be interpreted in a wider rather than narrower sense) should be eliminated. The Working Party took a clear view that direct participation in executions by doctors is unethical.

With regard to the provision of medical testimony in capital trials, the Working Party felt that testimony which contributed to determination of a death penalty posed major ethical problems, which it was unable to resolve satisfactorily. We have attempted to distinguish between valid medical opinion based on fact, and speculative pejorative hypothesizing which is not. In practical terms, however, such defining lines are not easily drawn.

The BMA has previously taken the view that it is not the role of the doctor to certify a prisoner fit for punishment. Equally, therefore, we see it as inappropriate for a doctor to enter into court speculation about whether a prisoner ought to be subject to corporal or capital punishment. There would be irony in opposing medical involvement in the administration of a few strokes of a cane but not opposing whatever processes end in the execution of a person. Moreover, presentation of medical evidence based on the type of hypothetical questions we have considered, rather than on an examination of the prisoner, is scientifically unacceptable. Nevertheless, the Working Party did not wish to preclude doctors responding to a request from a prisoner to give evidence on his or her behalf. It would be hard to guarantee that medical testimony offered in mitigation of an offence would never include an element of speculation of hypothesis. Logically, if such evidence, although intended to help the prisoner, fails to convince a court it may be held to be contributory to a death sentence being passed.

In practical terms we believe that it may be simpler to oppose capital punishment *per se* rather than attempt to define ways in which to eliminate medical participation in all phases of the process through which an individual is sentenced to death. At present, however, we recognize that there is no clear consensus within the profession on abolition. We believe, however, that the medical profession should work towards the objective of ending medical participation in those parts of the judicial process leading to execution.

Certification of death is a statutory requirement which is unaffected by the nature of the death though the process by which certification takes place (e.g. coroner's inquest) varies in different circumstances and jurisdictions. The Working Party had sympathy for the view that doctors should not certify an executed prisoner but felt that, provided the certification was carried out outside the immediate site of execution, it was consistent with medical ethics. However, doctors should not attend executions; they are not medical procedures and doctors should not contribute to the view that there is a legitimate role for a doctor during such a procedure.

Chapter 7

Hunger strikes and other human rights issues involving prisoners

A prisoner is potentially in a worse condition than the slave, because the slave is the property of someone whose interest is to keep his property in serviceable condition, whereas the prisoner is owned by nobody, unless it be the State which is ultimately responsible for his imprisonment. Consequently the condition of its prisons and its prisoners is no bad indication of the development of any society and its degree of civilisation.[1]

In addition to setting out to make an evaluation of medical involvement in torture and judicial punishments, the Working Party initially wished to give consideration to "the role of doctors in human rights abuses" and "extrajudicial punishments". We considered that this could cover a wide range of unethical situations ranging from abuses directed at prisoners to those directed against free citizens brought into conflict with the civil authority. Because the thrust of this report is directed towards those abuses involving individuals deprived of their liberty, we decided to confine discussion of other human rights issues to those related to prisoners.

Those prisoner-related ethical problems continuing to confront doctors include the voluntary total fast or hunger strike; intimate body searches; forcible taking of blood or tissue samples; withholding of medical care to prisoners; and involuntary medication. Other ethical and human rights issues such as medical treatment of asylum seekers, virginity testing, cultural surgical procedures (most importantly female circumcision), forcible sterilization, experiments on prisoners and trade in human organs will be briefly mentioned but were considered outside

---

1 Kenneth Ruch. Introduction to the 1929 Everyman edition of John Howard's *The State of the Prisons in England and Wales*. Cited in: Smith R. *Prison Health Care*. London: BMA, 1984, p.5.

the terms of reference of the Working Party; they deserve more attention than can be given here.

Hunger strikes and forcible feeding

Hunger strikes present the doctor with a complex and difficult moral problem which can at the most serious extreme resolve itself to a choice between respecting the prisoner's expressed will and perhaps watching him or her die a slow, distressing and avoidable death, or overriding the prisoner's expressed wish in order to preserve the prisoner's life. The techniques used to provide nourishment forcibly have often been most unpleasant. In February 1974 in an open letter to the BMA, the Action Committee Supporting Irish Prisoners described the techniques then used in Britain:

> They are forcibly fed in the following manner. Their mouths are forced open with a surgical instrument and a thick greased orange tube is pushed down their throats. A liquid mixture is then poured down and this is almost always followed by vomiting and nausea. The prisoners are held down by wardens.[2]

Doctors writing to the Association in 1974 added other details:

> The method used for forcible feeding has remained the same since the beginning of this century when suffragettes were fed in this way. Between the teeth a wooden block is placed, containing a hold through which a greased stomach tube is passed. This process is performed once or twice a day and may be repeated if vomiting occurs. Where resistance is encountered, a steel clamp is used to prise open the mouth, and several people may be required to hold the subject still.[3]

Such an aggressive and potentially dangerous approach to forcible feeding is not the only way in which feeding is accomplished. Where a prisoner does not resist physically, is sedated, or is too weak to resist, feeding by intravenous infusion can be carried out.

The political and psychological aspects of the hunger strike represent an additional complexity to the phenomenon. While the hunger strike which ends in fatality is a dramatic and tragic event it is far from typical. In 1981, for example, the year of the prolonged and fatal hunger strikes in Northern Ireland, there were 12 fatalities as a result

---

2   BMA archive.

3   *Ibid.*

of hunger strikes reported in Europe (including one in the USSR)[4]. Of these, ten occurred in Belfast.

By contrast, during the same year, in France alone there were at least 56 hunger strikes involving hundreds of prisoners undertaken in French prisons, with no fatalities[5]. It is difficult to know to what extent this relatively low level of fatality is due to the limited goals or commitment of hunger-strikers or to the forcible intervention by medical or other prison staff.

In general, hunger strikes are not carried out with the objective of the death of the hunger-striker. Indeed, a hunger strike usually ends well before serious injury is done due to an intended limitation of the fast, change of mind of the prisoner, persuasion by family, lawyer or prison officers, or capitulation in the face of pressure, including forcible feeding, from the authorities. In certain circumstances the death of one or more prisoners may have been anticipated in advance and may even have represented an element in a confrontation with a government, though this appears to be very rare.

In repressive societies where avenues for legitimate political protest are unavailable, the hunger strike assumes a quite important form of power for the prisoner. However, it is also the context in which the prisoner will be most likely to have his or her rights disregarded. This may mean that doctors are brought into the conflict, not so much to save the prisoner's life as a humanitarian endeavour but rather to inflict on the prisoner the will of the government. The example from Morocco recounted below is a stark example of this. When the World Medical Association set out to codify its policy on torture and other cruel, inhuman or degrading punishments in the early 1970s, it included the hunger strike in this procedure. This was in part a response to the political context in which some hunger strikes were being carried out in the 1970s and the use of forcible feeding as a repressive arm of the state. It was clear that in some countries, artificial forcible feeding was primarily administered as a government policy rather than being the outcome of a doctor's clinical judgement. The World Medical Association's 1975 Declaration of Tokyo included the following provision:

---

4   Duhamel O. Esquisse d'une typologie des grèves de la faim [Sketch of a typology of hunger strikes]. In: *La Grève de la Faim*. Paris: Economica, 1984. p.23. The information was drawn from an analysis of reports in the French daily *Le Monde*.

5   *Ibid.*, pp.36-40.

Where a prisoner refuses nourishment and is considered by the doctor as capable of forming an unimpaired and rational judgment concerning the consequences of such a voluntary refusal of nourishment, he or she shall not be fed artificially. The decision as to the capacity of the prisoner to form such a judgment should be confirmed by at least one other independent doctor. The consequences of the refusal of nourishment shall be explained by the doctor to the prisoner. [Art. 5]

This has been the clearest international statement by the medical profession on the subject of hunger strikes. While this paragraph can form the basis of a coherent policy towards hunger-strikers[6], it does not totally solve the problem, however, since there remains the question of the appropriate response in the absence of a prisoner's clearly expressed wish to fast to the point of death and in the situation where a prisoner has passed the point where an informed decision can be made. The WMA itself has suggested that doctors could feed hunger-strikers in the absence of consent in certain circumstances[7] and gave notice that it was continuing a discussion on the appropriate policy on the doctor and hunger strikes. In November 1991 at the World Medical Association annual assembly in Malta, a set of principles was adopted (see appendix).

The UK: evolution of policy

In the United Kingdom, the policy on the management of hunger strikes has evolved both in the political and medical spheres. With respect to government policy, there has been a progressive evolution in the attitude of the authorities towards hunger-strikers. Earlier in the century, those undertaking hunger strikes could have no illusions about the treatment they would receive and involuntary feeding was carried out in, from all accounts, a fairly brusque fashion[8]. The Prison Rules (1964) bound the prison medical officer in unspecific terms to care for the mental and physical health of the prisoner. Although nothing in the rules specifically justified force-feeding, the Home Office standing orders — Rule 17 (i) Prison Rules 1964: SI No. 388 — laid down the advisability of admission to the prison hospital for assessment of the need for compulsory artificial force-feeding.

---

6 Kalk WJ, Veriava Y. Hospital management of voluntary total fasting among political prisoners. *Lancet*, 1991; 337:660-2.

7 World Medical Association. News release. 3 June 1991.

8 For a review of the medicolegal issues see: Anon. The law and force-feeding. *British Medical Journal*, 1974; 2:737-8.

Even though in the 1960s there was to some degree a transition from strict forcible feeding to more prisoner-centred treatment, as late as the spring of 1974, young Irish prisoners held in Brixton prison were being forcibly fed throughout a hunger strike lasting from November 1973 to the summer of 1974. In January 1974, Mr Mark Carlisle, Minister of State at the Home Office, stated in the Commons that four men and two women were being artificially force-fed in prisons in England and Wales. The case of the Irish prisoners raised a furore within the medical profession in this country. Two of the prisoners, the Price sisters, issued proceedings against the Home Office challenging the right to force-feed in any case other than that where refusal of food arose from a medical or psychiatric illness. This led to the then Home Secretary, Roy Jenkins, stating in the House of Commons on 17 July 1974:

> The doctor's obligation is to the ethics of his profession and to his duty at common law; he is not required as a matter of prison practice to feed a prisoner artificially against the prisoner's will. Since there has been misunderstanding on this point, I think it is in the interests of prisoners, the medical profession and the public, that the procedures to be followed in future should leave no room for doubt.
>
> I am advised that the common law duty placed upon a person in charge of a prisoner is to take such steps as are reasonable in the circumstances of each case to preserve the health and the life of the prisoner. In making their decision in respect of any particular case they must have regard not merely to the dangers likely to flow from the prisoner's refusal of food, but also to those likely to flow from the practice of forced feeding itself, if it is resorted to, and particularly if it is resisted.
>
> Accordingly, the future practice should, in my view, be that if a prisoner persists in refusing to accept any form of nourishment, the medical officer should first satisfy himself that the prisoner's capacity for rational judgment is unimpaired by illness, mental or physical. If the medical officer is so satisfied he should seek confirmation of his opinion from an outside consultant. If the consultant confirms the opinion of the prison medical officer, the prisoner should be told that he will continue to receive medical supervision and advice and that food will be made available for him.
>
> He should be informed that he will be removed to the prison hospital if and when this is considered appropriate. But it should be made clear to him that there is no rule of prison practice which requires the prison medical officer to resort to artificial feeding (whether by tube or intravenously). Finally, he should be plainly and categorically warned that the consequent and inevitable deterioration in his health may be allowed to continue without medical intervention, unless he specifically requests it.
>
> I have discussed this subject with my Rt Hon Friends the Secretaries of State for Scotland and Northern Ireland, who have decided that the

procedures I have outlined will apply also in Scotland and Northern Ireland.[9]

This has remained the attitude of successive governments since that time. The BMA debated the issue intensively in 1974 and 1975[10] and was torn by the dilemma of wishing to preserve life while respecting the prisoner's wishes. It felt that doctors who had conscientious objections must be able to refrain from participating in force-feeding, and that no doctor should be pressurised by government policy. A letter to the *Lancet*[11] alleged that the doctor supervising the forced feeding of the two young women in Brixton prison had stated he had no desire to force-feed them, but was carrying out the orders of the Home Office. This gave grounds for concern and the BMA, in a statement issued in 1975 giving clarification for doctors on "medical aspects of interrogation and of artificial feeding of prisoners", cited the Home Secretary's statement quoted above. This paper also cited in full the statement of policy adopted at the 1974 ARM of the BMA, the essence of which was that, with regard to hunger strikes, "the final decision must be for [the prison medical officer] to make, and it is not for some outside person to seek to override the clinical judgment of the doctor by imposing his own decision upon the case in question"[12]. The BMA policy as set out in the 1981 *Handbook of Medical Ethics* continued to leave decisions on forcible feeding to the individual doctor, while drawing attention to the WMA's Declaration of Tokyo. In later pronouncements on the subject, the BMA again stressed the need to balance respect for the patient's autonomy with a need to act wherever possible in the prisoner's best interests.

In practice, the major political hunger strikes in the United Kingdom over the past 15 years have been managed essentially in a manner consistent with the policy embodied in article 5 of the Declaration of Tokyo. These included the hunger strikes of 1981 in Northern Ireland

---

9 *Hansard*; **877** col. 451, 1974.

10 See for example: BMA Central Ethical Committee. Ethical Statement: Artificial feeding of Prisoners. *British Medical Journal*, 1974; 3:52.

11 Moore M. Force-feeding of prisoners (letter) *Lancet*, 1974; i:1109.

12 *Statement by the British Medical Association upon the medical aspects of interrogation and of artificial feeding of prisoners*. January 1975. 6pp. The issue was of immediate relevance. In 1976, two IRA prisoners, Frank Stagg and Michael Gaughan, went on indefinite hunger strike. In contrast to the treatment of the Price sisters whose hunger strike continued for 200 days with forced feeding, the two men were not fed and they died while striking in English prisons for political status.

when first Bobby Sands, and later other members of the Provisional IRA (Irish Republican Army) and INLA (Irish National Liberation Army), fasted to death with the medical officers providing advice and medical supervision but respecting the prisoners' clearly-expressed wishes to continue their fast[13].

Experiences outside the UK

In other countries, hunger strikes remain a potent source of controversy and social conflict. Sixty members of the militant Spanish organization GRAPO (*Grupos de Resistencia Antifascista Primero de Octubre*) who, as a result of a change in policy in 1987 had been dispersed to different prisons in Spain, undertook hunger strikes in late 1989 to press for the right of all GRAPO prisoners to be held in the same prison. The strike occasioned much public debate about the ethical and legal implications of forced feeding. Judges in Madrid, Zaragoza and Valladolid became involved in polemic debate with local penal authorities. The former claimed that forced feeding of a conscious individual was contrary to Article 5 of the Spanish Constitution which prohibits inhuman or degrading treatments. Government ministers, however, shared the view of judges in six other cities[14] that the State has an overriding legal and moral obligation to maintain the health and lives of prisoners in its care[15]. The intentions of the prisoners were subject to lengthy philosophical analysis in national newspapers as it was argued by some that prisoners have a constitutional right to bring about their own death but no legal right to impose pressure on the authorities to change policies.

The dilemma quickly involved Spanish doctors. The Medical Council (*Consejo General de Médicos*) issued a circular which, although intended to state the ethical and legal position, does not appear to have been entirely helpful. It stated:

A doctor cannot impose a treatment contrary to the will of the patient, unless failure to do so would constitute a public health risk or when an emergency

---

13 For accounts of the hunger strike see Beresford D. *Ten Men Dead*. London: Grafton, 1987; O'Malley P. *Biting at the Grave: The Irish Hunger Strikes and the Politics of Despair*. Belfast: The Blackstaff Press, 1990.

14 The judges of Albacete, Murcia, Sevilla, Soria, Guadalajara and Valencia favoured forced feeding while the judge in Bilboa appeared to waver between both positions.

15 See, for example: Etica y derecho sin recetas. *El Pais*, 29 January 1990; Huelga de hambre y obligaciones del Estado. *El Pais*, 7 March 1990.

obliges the doctor to intervene to prevent death or irreversible damage. Such judgements can only and exclusively be made by doctors, or the medical team, in the exercise of their profession.

It went on to state:

When refusal of treatment may not be justified, the doctor is obliged to obey the order of the competent authority, whether judicial or administrative. The Penal Code only excludes compliance with such orders when to obey "constitutes a clear and manifest infraction of a legal principle" according to Article 369 of the Penal Code.[16]

Furthermore, the circular justified involuntary medical intervention in cases where the patient's life is at risk and the patient shows a clearly suicidal intention. At the same time, it enjoined doctors to "respect the patients' liberty" and urged patients to voluntarily modify their behaviour. A difficulty was that the circular itself was left open to interpretation, although *Consejo General* sources were quoted as interpreting it as a rejection of forced feeding in favour of persuasion of the conscious patient, treatment only being forcibly applied when the patient loses consciousness[17]. This led to doctors accusing the judges of "washing their hands of a politically difficult problem by making it a medical dilemma"[18].

At the end of January 1990, after two months' strike, the health of some of the prisoners was approaching a critical stage. In mid-February 1990, authorities in Zaragoza and Madrid ordered that prisoners be forcibly fed, despite the opposition of judges. When the three Zaragoza prisoners were taken to hospital, Dr José Ramon Muñoz, head of the nutrition unit, decided as a matter of conscience that he could not let the three die and so commenced involuntary feeding. This persuaded the judge in Zaragoza to approve forcible feeding.

On 27 March 1990, Dr Muñoz was shot dead by two members of GRAPO[19]. On 25 May 1990, one of the hunger-strikers died. Some of the prisoners gave up their fast in June 1990. However, with the legal

---

16 Dos presos de los GRAPO se quitan los tubos de alimentación forzosa [Two GRAPO prisoners give up forcible feeding]. *El Pais*. January 1990.

17 *Ibid.*

18 Statement from the Director of the Basurto Civil Hospital, Bilbao reported in *El Pais, ibid.*

19 *Le Monde*, 29 March 1990.

backing of the constitutional court in July 1990, the policy of forced feeding continued[20]. The strike finished in early 1991.

Across the straits of Gibraltar in Morocco, another hunger strike was undertaken between mid-1985 and August 1991. Two prisoners, Hassan Aharrat and Noureddine Jouhari, were forcibly fed via nasogastric tube from the time they were first admitted to Averroes Hospital in Casablanca in August 1985 in the second month of their strike, until August 1991, when they were released. This hunger strike and another, started in Rabat in June 1989, were undertaken in protest at inadequate medical treatment for prisoners who had been tortured. The two Casablanca prisoners are believed to have been held separately and incommunicado in the basement of Averroes Hospital, a university teaching hospital. According to reports[21], both men were held bound to their beds and left unwashed; they were kept sedated; their clothing and bedding was changed only a couple of times a year as was the tubing used to feed them. They were medically neglected; their medical care was left in the hands of guards who were supervised by two professors of medicine. Doctors and nurses who protested against this were brutally repressed and some staff were dismissed The prisoners had not seen their families since 1985 and had equally been denied access to lawyers throughout the period of the hunger strike[22]. The two men were among 40 political prisoners who were freed on 16 August 1991 following a royal amnesty[23].

Other hunger strikers in Rabat who started to refuse food in June 1989 and finished their hunger strike in February 1990 were reported to be in a poor state several months after ending their protest. One of their number, Chbada Abdelhaq, died on the 64th day of his hunger strike. In these latter cases, it is not clear what precise role was being played by doctors though it is clear in the case of Averroes Hospital that whatever medical advice was given it was apparently not as a result of medical examinations. Moreover, certain parts of the hospital appear to be used as a prison. The BMA wrote in 1989 about these serious cases

---

20 Interior y justicia, enfrentados por la huelga de hambre de los grapos. *Interviu*, 16-22 July 1990, pp.24-9.

21 See for example: Raat A-M. Hunger strikes in Morocco. *Lancet*, 1989; ii:982; Amnesty International. *Medical concern: continuing hunger strike, Morocco*. AI Index: MDE 29/21/90, 7 November 1990.

22 Amnesty International. *Medical concern: prolonged hunger strike, Morocco*. AI Index: MDE 29/07/89, 14 September 1989.

23 Amnesty International. *Morocco: forty political prisoners freed*. AI Index: NWS 11/30/91 addendum, 19 August 1991.

to the hospital, the *Ordre des Médecins* (medical association) and the *Conseil National de Médecine* (medical council) but received no reply to any of its letters.

In a report published in the *Lancet* in March 1991, doctors at Johannesburg Hospital described the way in which they had implemented Article 5 of the Declaration of Tokyo in their care of prisoners, held under the State of Emergency Regulations and the Internal Security Act, who were admitted to the hospital during 1989 while undertaking hunger strikes. Fifteen prisoners held under section 29 of the ISA (which permits indefinite detention without trial) were admitted to hospital after 10-12 days of voluntary total fasting (VTF). Medical and nursing staff decided to regard the prisoners as ordinary patients as far as possible and to give treatment consistent with the Declaration of Tokyo. This led to three treatment principles:

> First, the principle of full patient participation and consent in all clinical decision was applied. Second, the ethical provisions with respect to hunger strike (article 5 of the Declaration) and the consequences of VTF were explained objectively. The patients were not pressurised to end their fast, and the confidentiality of all discussion was emphasised. Thirdly, it was decided to try to prevent police interference in patient care.[24]

Police guards were present at all times and some behaved in a manner which caused considerable friction with staff. Police interference increased over time: doctor-patient discussions were deemed to be not privileged and a policeman attended such discussions (although this practice was rescinded after vigorous protest); police attempted to restrict nursing contact with patients who were also deprived of personal privacy; some of the hunger-strikers were chained to their beds. Medical staff protested at these procedures which were subsequently ended. Kalk and Veriava assert that the "legal conditions of detention without trial in South Africa are in conflict with medical ethics [which] have been subverted by the legalisation of unacceptable, unethical practices" and adopted a policy of refusing to allow their patients to be returned to the conditions which provoked their hunger strikes.

Recently, a diverse range of political, medical and human rights bodies in South Africa provisionally agreed a set of protocols for the medical management of hunger-strikers. These protocols included the following provisions:

---

24 Kalk WJ, Veriava Y. Hospital management of voluntary total fasting among political prisoners. *Lancet*, 1991; **337**:660-2.

All hunger strikers who have been on hunger strike for longer than two
(2) weeks or who have lost more that 10% of their original body weight,
must be hospitalized, with their consent, in non-prison hospitals. Consent
to hospitalization does not imply consent to other forms of treatment.
This does not preclude earlier hospitalisation of hunger strikers for other
medical reasons.

Additionally, there was a section relating to ethical codes which were
to include the following provisions:

- no medical personnel may apply pressure of any sort on the
  hunger-striker to suspend the hunger strike although the hunger-
  striker must be professionally informed of the medical
  consequences of hunger strike.
- medical care or treatment must be rendered to hunger-strikers
  unconditionally.
- hunger-strikers have the right to an independent second
  professional opinion.
- the hunger-striker will not be force-fed.
- the hunger-striker should be encouraged to make a living will
  stating his/her wishes with regard to treatment once they are unable
  to make such decision.[25]

The hunger strike is without doubt a difficult issue for doctors and other
health personnel. Those who carry them out for political reasons are
usually young, committed people who, in other circumstances, would
have everything to live for[26]. To watch such a person steadily
deteriorate to the point of death, over perhaps a two-month period, must
represent a stressful experience for medical and nursing staff. And yet,
at least in those cases where the prisoner has clearly expressed a wish

---

25 Communication from the National Medical and Dental Association of South
Africa (NAMDA), June 1991. Other organizations agreeing to the protocol were:
the Medical Association of South Africa, the South African Health Workers
Congress, the Organization for Appropriate Social Services in South Africa, the
African National Congress, and the Human Rights Commission, as well as the
government departments of Health, Justice, Law and Order and Correctional
Services. While the "living will" concept in the context of South African hunger
strikes may be a positive development, the coercion applying in other countries may
render a living will valueless without the doctor being able to confirm the prisoner's
wishes directly with the prisoner (where they are conscious).

26 Though most hunger-strikes are not undertaken for political reasons, but rather
for personal protest. O'Connor A, Johnson-Sabine E. Hunger strikers. *Medicine,
Science and Law*, 1988; **28**:62-4.

to carry out such a hunger strike, the doctor's respect for the decision reflects acceptance of the prisoner's autonomy and right to accept or refuse medical care. A hunger strike to death cannot be equated with suicide. The latter, in its most literal sense, represents a desire or depressed compulsion to end life. As a general rule, prisoners who refuse food do not do so in order to end their life but rather to put pressure on the authorities to change a policy. They *may* die as a result of the hunger strike but this is not its primary objective in most cases[27].

All this is clear in the case of prisoners able to express their choice before and during the hunger strike and where there is continuity in medical supervision. In such circumstances, the Working Party felt that the present policy as set out by the BMA and embodied in the Declaration of Tokyo was correct. However, the Working Party noted that there are countries where practice is to feed without consent when the prisoner loses consciousness and is not in a position to express a view at the time. This suggests that there is a need to investigate the legal standing of "living wills" in this context, something we will not attempt to do here.

There are circumstances where a hunger strike poses serious moral dilemmas. Two will be mentioned here. The first occurs when a prisoner is brought to a doctor in a comatose state and the doctor is unable to determine (or is unable to find out) the wishes of the prisoner. In such a hypothetical circumstance, we believe that the doctor ought to respond in the usual way when confronted by a seriously ill and unconscious patient who cannot be questioned. Treatment should be instituted to save the prisoner's life and to enable him or her, once resuscitated and able to communicate again, to inform the doctor of his or her wishes.

The second occurs when the doctor is faced with knowledge of the deteriorating prisoner's wishes to proceed with the hunger strike while the prisoner's family's actively-expressed wish is to preserve his or her life. This could be particularly poignant where there is discussion of an

---

27 It may be useful here to distinguish two other forms of food refusal which are of a different nature to the hunger strike. The first is reactive food refusal — the short-lived refusal of food in a fit of pique which will come to a natural end without intervention. The second is that carried out by a determined food refuser — a prisoner perhaps in an impossible position with no sense of a future. This prisoner who may not have been incompetent at the start may slip into a severe depression and undertake a form of deliberate self-inflicted suffering with the ultimate intent of dying. This type of case is rarer than the reactive food refuser and is distinctly different to the determined hunger-striker who seeks change rather than death.

end to a politically-organized or group-supported mass hunger strike and where the doctor is aware that by the time the hunger strike is called off, one or more hunger-strikers may be dead. In such a case we believe the doctor must balance respect for the prisoner's autonomy with developments since the prisoner's decision was made and in particular since the prisoner lost the capacity to express a clear, informed opinion. In cases where the original cause of the hunger strike has been resolved in agreement with the prisoner's view, treatment should be instigated immediately.

Also stemming from group hunger strikes is the problematic judgment which the doctor must make as to when the individual prisoner is genuinely and freely deciding to continue a strike and when he or she is continuing it due to irresistible group pressure[28]. If the prisoner appears to the doctor to be likely to want to give up the hunger strike but cannot do so in the presence of striking comrades, should the doctor request that the prisoner be moved in order to ease the pressure and allow him or her to make a free choice? Given that such a move may be seen as a deliberate attempt to divide the strikers and thus break the strike, such a decision should be made with the utmost sensitivity to the prisoner's best interests. One way of helping to determine the prisoner's wishes could be the introduction of a scheme which applies in the Netherlands where "doctors of confidence" are made available to striking prisoners allowing them direct contact with doctors outside the prison system. In many countries, however, the reality is that doctors will have to make such decisions on their own and will need the clearest available guidance.

During 1991, the WMA discussed the ethical response to hunger-strikers. The detailed discussion document did not meet the perceived need expressed during discussions in the WMA Ethics committee, and subsequently a revised statement of WMA policy was adopted by the general assembly of the WMA at its annual meeting in Malta. This is included in the appendices.

Forcible medication for non-medical reasons

The Working Party received allegations that prisoners in several countries were forcibly administered psychotropic drugs for non-medical

---

28 See O'Malley P. *Biting at the Grave: The Irish Hunger Strikes and the Politics of Despair, op. cit.* for an account of the complexity of the group/individual/family interplay during the 1981 strike.

purposes and that such drugs either had significant deleterious side-effects or gave rise to fears that they would have such side-effects.

Well-known examples of this in non-democratic countries include adminstration of chlorpromazine or haloperidol in the former USSR to prisoners held in psychiatric hospitals for political reasons; these abuses were discussed in the 1986 BMA report. Since that time, there have been both positive and negative changes in the USSR/CIS which have been discussed in Chapter 5.

Another case was the administration of psychoactive drugs to prisoners held in Libertad prison in Uruguay during the period of military dictatorship in that country (1972-83)[29]. In this case, psychiatrists prescribed and administered medication, often without appearing to adequately examine the prisoner. Moreover, neuroleptics were given without accompanying anti-Parkinsonian medication. This contributed to a feeling within the prison that there was a plan or system to psychologically dismantle the prisoners[30].

However, it is not only in non-democratic states where allegations of misuse of drugs are made. In Sweden in 1982, a complaint was made to the Swedish Medical Association (SMA) that medical personnel had administered tranquillizers to some of 24 Chileans who were being forcibly deported back to Chile after being refused asylum. It was alleged that a nurse administered drugs provided by a police doctor. During the flight, two of the deportees were given haloperidol in tea without their knowledge by a nurse travelling on the plane. The central committee of the SMA concluded that medical ethics had been breached and recommended that:

> Doctors should never, themselves or through instructions of others, collaborate in forced medication of persons who are not mentally ill or of patients who are unable, for other reasons, to give their consent. Medication should always be in the patient's own interest and not for the attainment of political objectives or those of the police.
>
> Persons who are not mentally ill must not be medicated "surreptitiously", i.e. be given medicine orally or in other ways without having been informed thereof and without having given their consent.[31]

---

29 Bloche M.G. *Uruguay's military physicians: Cogs in a System of State Terror.* Washington: AAAS, 1987; *Mental health aspects of political imprisonment in Uruguay.* Amnesty International, AI Index: AMR 52/18/83, 7 June 1983.

30 *Ibid.*; Weschler L. *A Miracle, A Universe: Settling Accounts with Torturers.* New York: Pantheon, 1990, pp.124-38.

31 Cited in: Rasmussen OV. Medical Aspects of Torture. *Danish Medical Bulletin*, 1990; **37** Supplement 1:83.

In Canada, reports in 1990 that deportees were being forcibly sedated prior to expulsion[32] led to protests from medical and refugee support groups. A review of all cases of medically-accompanied deportations in 1989 and 1990 by the Canadian immigration minister, Mrs Barbara McDougall, resulted in guidelines on the subject of the sedation of deportees. The two guiding principles were the following:

> under no circumstance will any person be taken to a physician solely for the purpose of that person being placed under sedation for removal from Canada;
> where a person has been taken to a physician for some other legitimate medical reason, the physician may address the question of sedation for removal as a secondary issue. If the physician decides to prescribe medication, the person concerned must be asked if he or she wishes to take such medication, and if not, no medication is to be given. (The only exception to this is in ... psychiatric cases...).[33]

More commonly, however, allegations are made about forcible use of drugs on prisoners and other detainees. American prisoners have alleged that they have been forcibly medicated in the absence of medical reasons[34]. The circumstances in which prisoners can be medicated against their will in the US are not subject to uniform procedures[35]. Each state has its own way of proceeding and in some states there appear to be no clearly defined procedures at all. The court decision which appears to set a standard in this area is the US Supreme Court decision in *Washington v. Harper*, 1990. Walter Harper had been in Washington state prisons since 1976, convicted of robbery. After four years imprisonment, during which time he voluntarily accepted antipsychotic medication, he was released on parole. During his parole period he twice was hospitalized and his parole was ended when he

---

32 *Globe and Mail* [Toronto], 9,10 May 1990.

33 Employment and Immigration Canada. Operations Memorandum: Medical escorts. OM number IE 306. 18 June 1990.

34 See, for example, *Sunday Punch* [Phoenix], 18 March 1990, p.3. A convicted bank robber, Dannie Martin, responded to a US Supreme Court decision in *Washington v. Harper* permitting involuntary medication, with a lengthy article. Whether or not he can be regarded as informed, the types of allegations he makes persist; he stated the following: "It's true that some convicts need to be medicated, but we have seen others who don't need the drugs being forced to take them by incompetent and tyrannical bureaucrats ....It is our observation that psychotropic drugs are ... used to quell what prison officials view as 'troublesome' prisoners".

35 Appelbaum PS. The right to refuse treatment with anti-psychotic medications: retrospect and prospect. *American Journal of Psychiatry*, 1988; **145**:413-19.

assaulted two nurses. He was then sent to a special psychiatric unit run by the Department of Corrections. He subsequently refused medication at this centre and procedures were initiated to commence involuntary medication. Harper appeared before a board composed of a psychiatrist, a psychologist and the associate superintendent of the psychiatric centre. The panel found that Harper met the civil commitment criteria for involuntary medication and thus approved involuntary medication, a finding which was eventually appealed all the way to the US Supreme Court. The Court review provoked great interest and led the American Psychiatric Association to contribute an *amicus curiae* brief in favour of the Washington procedure and the American Psychological Association to submit an *amicus* brief in favour of Mr Harper.

In *Washington v. Harper*, the Supreme Court ruled that the procedure for reviewing decisions to forcibly medicate which operated in the Washington State penal service was not unconstitutional[36]. For federal prisoners the decision is definitive. According to Appelbaum:

> the Constitution will allow even competent inmates to be treated against their will if they are dangerous to themselves or others (a standard likely to be construed broadly) and if treatment would be in their interests. Judges need not be involved in the decision."[37]

However, as most prisoners are covered by state rather than federal regulations, the effect of this on the majority remains to be seen. In any event, recent experience suggests that the majority of proposed decisions to forcibly medicate in jurisdictions with review procedures are supported by the review panel[38].

Persistent allegations of non-medical use of psychotropic drugs have also been made in the southern German state of Bavaria where there have been a number of press reports that prisoners held in the prison at Straubing are medicated with neuroleptics unnecessarily, sometimes by force[39].

---

36 Appelbaum PS. Washington v. Harper: Prisoners' rights to refuse anti-psychotic medication. *Hospital and Community Psychiatry*, 1990; **41**:731-2.

37 *Ibid.*

38 Appelbaum PS. The right to refuse treatment with anti-psychotic medications: retrospect and prospect. *Op. cit.*

39 See, for example: Verzweifelte Häftlinge in der "Hölle von Straubing" [Desperate prisoners in the "hell of Straubing".] *Süddeutsche Zeitung*, 7/8 April 1990, p.26.

While there has apparently been no successful legal action taken to resolve the allegations made in Bavaria, a case in Austria which was taken to the European Commission on Human Rights throws some light on the legal issues involved. The applicant, a Hungarian refugee resident in Austria, was detained between 1972 and 1984, as a result of a series of criminal convictions. According to the Commission report:

> During his detention in various prisons [during the early years of his imprisonment] the applicant was found to be a difficult prisoner, mainly because he addressed numerous petitions and complaints to various authorities concerning his allegedly wrongful convictions and his treatment in prison.[40]

Subsequently, he was diagnosed as suffering *paranoia querulans* and declared to lack legal capacity. In 1978 he was declared not responsible for his acts; it was asserted that his presence at a further trial could be harmful to his health and it was recommended by the court that he be sent to an institution for "mentally deranged offenders" from where he was sent to Vienna psychiatric hospital after commencing a hunger strike on 2 August 1979. He remained in the hospital until release in 1984.

The prisoner was given Taractan and Dapotum depot in December 1977 which he said was against his will. Six weeks after commencing his hunger strike in August 1979 he was ordered by the hospital department director to be fed involuntarily under the Hospitals Act. On 14 and 15 September 1979 he was given Taractan against his will and fed by infusion. On 17 September he was given Sordinol depot. Ten days later he stopped his hunger strike only to recommence it on 26 November 1979. On 13 December he agreed to feeding once a day through a tube. A month later, on 14 January 1978, it was decided in view of his deteriorating condition, to forcibly medicate the prisoner in order to feed him by infusion.

The following day he was forcible medicated though the circumstances of this medication were the subject of dispute. The government stated that he caused damage to the cell door and was armed with a club. An emergency squad was called in to overwhelm him. The prisoner claimed that he was asked by an officer in a helmet and gas mask whether he would agree to medication. On his refusal,

---

40 European Commission of Human Rights. Application No. 10533/83. *Istvan Herczegfalvy against Austria*. Report of the Commission, adopted 1 March 1991. Strasbourg: Council of Europe.

three tear gas grenades were thrown into his cell and he was subsequently attacked by ten emergency squad officers. He was then sent to an intensive care unit.

He was kept fettered more or less continuously for the next month during which he was given neuroleptic treatment. Over the ensuing period his medication was progressively lessened and eventually he was released in 1984.

In its report on the case, the European Commission of Human Rights addressed, among other aspects, the question of whether the applicant's treatment was in breach of article 3 of the European Convention prohibiting torture or cruel, inhuman or degrading treatment or punishment. With regard to the medical treatment itself:

> the Commission accept[ed] the Government's view which is supported by medical evidence. It appears that the treatment given to the applicant could reasonably be considered to be justified by medical considerations. The applicant's compulsory medical treatment was therefore not as such contrary to Article 3.[41]

However it concluded that:

> it is nevertheless doubtful whether in view of the applicant's reaction on 15 January 1980 it was really necessary to insist on the immediate administration of his compulsory treatment and apply massive force to this end.... [T]he use of force seems to have contributed to the applicant's state of agitation and his complete physical breakdown. ...
> Even if the fettering may have been unavoidable in order to secure his effective treatment, the manner in which it was carried out and the period during which it was maintained appear disproportionate. ...
> As to the applicant's compulsory feeding, the Commission considers that it could reasonably be regarded as necessary both in September and again in December 1979.[42]

The Commission concluded that "in particular during the period following the incident of 15 January 1980 the applicant's compulsory medical treatment and the way in which it was administered, combined with his artificial feeding and isolation, amounted to inhuman and degrading treatment"[43].

---

41 *Ibid.*, para. 244.

42 *Ibid.*, paras. 247-9.

43 *Ibid.*, para. 254.

The involuntary medication of prisoners is an issue which is simple to address in principle but undoubtedly more complex in reality. There is widespread agreement that medication should only be administered to a prisoner (or anyone else for that matter) with that person's consent or in limited and defined situations where informed consent cannot be given for different reasons[44]. In practice, in a prison environment, certainly in the UK and undoubtedly elsewhere, prisons are full of inmates ranging from the mentally sound to the frankly mentally ill[45]. When a prisoner is competent, the degree of voluntariness with which he can be said to acquiesce to treatment may be questioned. In the English case of *Freeman v Home Office*[46], life prisoner David Freeman alleged he had not consented to the administration of drugs; rather he had "actively resisted it, but was overcome forcibly by [a] medical officer and/or prison officers". Mr Louis Blom-Cooper QC, Counsel for the plaintiff, argued that it is impossible within the prison context for free and voluntary consent to exist between a prisoner and a prison medical officer. He reasoned that the prison medical officer is not merely a doctor, but a prison officer within the meaning of the Prison Rules and accordingly is a person who can influence a prisoner's life and his prospects of release on licence. There must inevitably be an atmosphere of constraint upon an inmate in such circumstances. However, the appeal court judge concurred with an earlier ruling that:

> where, in a prison setting, a doctor has the power to influence a prisoner's situation and prospects a court must be alive to the risk that what may appear, on the face of it, to be a real consent is not in fact so.[47]

Prisons also may have highly aggressive and anti-social inmates who pose serious management problems to prison staff. Such inmates, though

---

44 These include reasons of age (where consent would be given by a parent or guardian), unconsciousness (where emergency services would act with implied consent until actual consent could be given or denied), or mental disability due to mental handicap or mental illness to the extent that competence to consent has been judged not to exist.

45 Smith R. *Prison medicine*. London: British Medical Association, 1984; Gunn J, Maden A, Swinton M. Treatment needs of prisoners with psychiatric disorders. *British Medical Journal*, 1991; 303:338-41.

46 Brief details of the case of *Freeman v Home Office* (1984) QB 524, (1983) 1 All ER 1036, CA are given in: Kennedy I, Grubb A. *Medical Law: Text and Materials*. London: Butterworths, 1989, p.283.

47 *Ibid.*, p.875.

not seriously mentally ill, may provoke staff to request medical officers to use medication to bring the inmates under control[48]. Whether the medical officers accede to such requests should depend on the medical evaluation of the prisoner involved, taking into account the nature of the prisoner's mental state, his or her competence to consent to treatment and the prisoner's best interests.

Where long-term treatment is envisaged and the prisoner persistently refuses consent, there seems a strong argument for a review of the proposed treatment by, at a minimum, an independent physician or psychiatrist (as appropriate). In conjunction with this review of the proposed treatment, there should be a regular independent review during the course of involuntary treatment, and the prisoner should have the right to appeal to a review panel as recommended in the new UN principles for the protection of the mentally ill[49]. By setting out clear and workable protection and review procedures, it should be possible to avoid the misuse of drugs for punitive purposes and also to avoid the situation where the doctor is reluctant, on political grounds, to use drugs in the absence of consent in circumstances where there are real medical indications for such use.

Withholding medical care

The deliberate withholding of medical care for reasons other than contraindications or lack of availability of medicines could, *in extremis*, represent cruel, inhuman or degrading treatment. Amnesty International gives examples of behaviour by doctors which contravenes the most basic notions of ethics. For example:

a prisoner held in Kars prison in Turkey alleged that in 1984 he developed sores on his feet which the prison doctor responded to

---

48 In 1985 a contributor to a Prison Reform Trust book stated that: "It would appear that there is evidence that drugs are, at least sometimes, used for disciplinary rather than therapeutic reasons. No doubt such allegations will continue to be denied, but the evidence, though limited, speaks otherwise. It also appears that the use of drugs [in English prisons] is less prevalent than previously. It would also appear that this reduction in the use of drugs has been a direct result of agitation by certain groups of individuals and, but for that agitation, would not have occurred." Dr Tony Whitehead, cited in Sim J. *Medical Power in Prisons: The Prison Medical Service in England, 1774-1989*. Buckingham: Open University Press, 1990, p.114.

49 *Principles for the Protection of Persons with Mental Illness and for the Improvement of Mental Health Care*. UN General Assembly Resolution 46/119. Adopted 17 December 1991.

unsympathetically. When these sores worsened, he was prescribed a salve and though he eventually could not walk unaided he was not recommended for a hospital visit. After complaining about the doctor's behaviour, the prisoner was confronted by the doctor who ordered guards to beat him. When he was eventually transferred to hospital he had developed gangrene and had first his toes and later his foot, amputated".[50]

In South Africa, the record of the doctor placing the interests of the security forces before those of his or her patients is well-documented. The Biko affair, which stained the ethical reputation of South African medicine for a decade from the time of Biko's death in 1977, continues to be discussed[51]. Other cases appear to have occurred regularly since. For example, in 1983 Marcus Thabo Motaung was shot three times in the groin during arrest by police. He was taken to a district surgeon, Dr Snyman, who administered pain killers. Dr Snyman later told the Pretoria Supreme Court during Mr Motaung's trial for treason that she thought it more important for him to assist the police than to have immediate access to medical care. He was denied hospital treatment for two days as a result[52].

An Amnesty International report on women and human rights cites several cases where female prisoners were denied adequate treatment, sometimes with the apparent acquiescence of doctors. For example, a Moroccan woman wrote from prison that many fellow prisoners were suffering disorders resulting from torture. She alleged that:

> The prison authorities don't do anything to help us. We haven't even seen any medical specialists except for the physician of the prison.... His examination consisted of a single question, "Where does it hurt?" If you

---

50 Amnesty International. *Involvement of medical personnel in abuses against detainees and prisoners.* AI Index: ACT 75/08/90, November 1990, p.23.

51 Lee NC. Biko revisited [editorial]. *South African Medical Journal*, 1991; 79:635-6. The *New York Times* reported on 24 October 1991 that Dr Benjamin Tucker, one of Biko's doctors, had been readmitted to medical practice after apologising to the South African Medical and Dental Council for his actions. It quoted Tucker as saying: "I had become too closely identified with the interest of the organs of the state, especially the police force, with which I dealt practically on a daily basis. In the circumstances of Mr. Biko's case, I too readily accepted the decisions of the Security Police, without safeguarding the interests of my patient."

52 See Rayner M. *Turning a Blind Eye? Medical Accountability and the Prevention of Torture in South Africa.* Washington: American Association for the Advancement of Science, 1987, note 96, p.48. Motaung was one of three men hanged for treason in 1983, the first executions for treason in South Africa for more than 70 years.

do get a prescription, you face another problem: getting the medication.[53]

In some cases even the most minimal aid is withheld. A woman who was arrested in January 1986 in the Indian state of Gujarat was immediately sexually humiliated by the arresting police and later raped. At the police station she was again assaulted, including by the insertion of a bamboo into her vagina, causing profuse bleeding. Two days later she was taken to another police station where doctors apparently refused to examine her without receiving orders from the chief of police. An official investigation later found that a number of people, including doctors, had participated in the rape or in the cover-up.[54]

In several countries prisoners are chained to their beds while held in hospitals. For example, a Burmese medical student told a delegation from the US organization, Physicians for Human Rights, that he had seen two seriously wounded students shackled by the ankle to their hospital beds following demonstrations in March 1988. One of them died three weeks later from sepsis. Military interference in the running of health services was widely reported at the time[55].

Prisoners appear to be seriously neglected in many countries. Significant malnutrition and disease was reported in a study of prisoners seen in a provincial Nigerian hospital, leading the authors to suggest that "malnutrition [in prisoners] might ... be alarmingly common and severe in the developing world"[56]. In Malawi, prisoners also suffer serious nutritional disorders; one survey showed that more than half of prisoners screened had eye changes secondary to vitamin A deficiency, caused by the restricted and poor-quality diet[57].

Such structural inadequacies pose real problems for doctors who, by themselves, cannot overcome the effects of policies maintained by managers of the prison system. They can protest however.

---

53 Amnesty International. *Women in the Front Line: human rights violations against women*. London: AI Publications, 1991, p.28.

54 *Ibid.*, p.19

55 Hu H, U Kyaw Win, Arnison ND. Burma: health and human rights. *Lancet*, 1991; **337**:1335-6.

56 Olubodun JOB, Jaiyesimi AEA, Fakoya EA, Olasode OA. Malnutrition in prisoners admitted to a medical ward in a developing community. *British Medical Journal*, 1991; **303**:693-4.

57 Reeve PA. Prisoners and doctors. *British Medical Journal*, 1990; **300**:470.

Forcible examination of prisoners

Forcible non-medical examinations of the prisoner have an obvious potential to distress and humiliate. The British Medical Association has maintained that no forcible examination of prisoners should be carried out by doctors solely as part of government policy and contrary to the prisoner's interests (see below). Security is the reason usually advanced for the practices of strip searching (i.e., requiring a person to undress to partial or complete nakedness) and intimate body searches (i.e., internal examination to determine whether objects have been secreted in the vagina or rectum), though such examinations are also practised to allow the gathering of evidence for prosecution.

These are not medical examinations, though there may be circumstances where the individual concerned has put his or her life at risk through, for example, swallowing potentially lethal drugs. While there is, at the time of writing, no internationally-agreed ethical norm on such searches[58], individual medical associations have their own standards. In 1973, the BMA pledged the support of the British medical profession to colleagues in West Germany who were taking a principled stand against the West German government on the issue of forcible examination of prisoners. In a *British Medical Journal* editorial the Association stated:

> Whatever the law may command in our respective countries, we share the same ethical tradition in medicine, and the forcible examination of a person is contrary to it and the fact that the person is a prisoner would aggravate the offence.[59]

Later, in response to the introduction of the 1984 *Police and Criminal Evidence Act*, the BMA drew up guidelines to assist doctors in making a decision about whether or not to comply with requests by police officers to carry out intimate body searches of detainees. However, stronger recommendations were made by the 1988 ARM, which adopted a policy that doctors should not perform intimate body searches without the subject's consent. This remains the published policy of the Association.

---

58 The World Medical Association tried in 1991 to establish guidelines for such practices. However, following discussions at the Ethics Committee in May 1991 and at the WMA Assembly in November 1991, the draft document was withdrawn, and discussion deferred until 1992.

59 Anon. Forcible examination. *British Medical Journal*, 1973; 3:466.

In democratic countries such as the USA and the UK, there have been allegations that female prisoners in particular have been subjected to humiliation in the form of strip or intimate body searches. The introduction of strip searching in Armagh women's prison in 1982 led to a campaign for its abolition and to various official and unofficial enquiries into the practice[60]. In the USA, the special High Security Unit at Lexington, Kentucky created considerable controversy because of its oppressive conditions. One of the conditions which stimulated protest was the practice of "unacceptable strip searching". This was carried out systematically on the handful of women held there every time they went to the recreation yard:

> despite the fact that no more than one prisoner [subsequently two] could use the yard at any one time; that recreation was limited to one hour per day...; that the yard was subject to TV surveillance; that a guard was always in the yard during use; and that the yard could not be used when any workman or prisoner from the main yard was close....[61]

The Lexington HSU was subsequently closed after a court case brought by some of the prisoners held there.

Intimate body searches are an exceptional measure which ostensibly appear to be carried out solely for reasons of security. There is no apparent reason for the involvement of medical personnel though it is possible to envisage circumstances where a prisoner could *request* examination by a doctor rather than a prison officer. These circumstances could include the existence of medical problems which the prisoner either believes would require medical skills or wants to keep confidential, or a feeling that there would be less humiliation in an examination by a doctor.

The forcible taking of blood or tissue samples

At present in Britain, a person in custody is not obliged to submit to medical treatment or to provide specimens for forensic examination.

---

60 For a cautious review of the issues see: Standing Advisory Commission on Human Rights. *Searching of women prisoners in Northern Ireland*. Belfast: SAC, 9 December 1986. For a briefer review of the practice in the whole UK see: The Howard League. *Strip Searching in UK Prisons*. London: Howard League for Penal Reform, November 1989. Both suggest the reform of strip searching rather than its abolition.

61 Amnesty International. *United States of America: the High Security Unit, Lexington Federal Prison, Kentucky*, AI Index: AMR 51/34/88, August 1988. Appendix 4.6, pp.7-8. [Report to AI by Rod Morgan.]

There have been suggestions from the Home Office in recent years that doctors should have a role in obtaining body samples to aid police investigations in cases where the prisoner does not willingly consent. Techniques such as DNA profiling (genetic fingerprinting) would allow for some suspects to be exonerated and, as such, represents a useful medical procedure in the interests of the detained person. Nevertheless, it is the BMA's view that if the prisoner refused for any reason to provide blood or tissue cells for examination after the procedure has been explained to him/her, police surgeons should not participate in the forcible extraction of such material.

The growing pandemic of HIV/AIDS has led to calls for compulsory measures of all sorts, including blood tests. Such compulsory tests are not justified on medical grounds[62].

Asylum seekers

Although not strictly within its remit, the Working Party was particularly concerned about the plight of asylum seekers who flee their own countries after experiencing harassment, torture or political imprisonment. We were distressed to hear about three successful suicides and many unsuccessful suicide attempts which were made by asylum seekers held in detention in Britain during the period 1987-1990. Many of those who seek refuge in the UK arrive in an understandably depressed or anxious state, and many have a limited command of the English language. Asylum seekers are often detained while assessment is made of their status as refugees and this detention may compound any psychological problems already in existence. The Working Party wished to bring attention to the dilemmas faced by doctors working with asylum seekers. These dilemmas are related to those of doctors working with tortured prisoners — where intervention may benefit the prisoner in the short-term, while acting against his interests in the longer term.

Doctors who treat asylum seekers for injuries caused by torture may, for the best of reasons, diminish the signs of maltreatment. Clear evidence of torture gives a strong case for asylum, and treatment which helps healing may increase the chances of the person being returned to a hazardous situation. Doctors should therefore pay attention to recording any injuries they find in a person seeking asylum.

---

62 Sieghart P. *AIDS and Human Rights: a UK Perspective*. London: BMA Foundation for AIDS, 1989; *Report of an International Consultation on AIDS and Human Rights; Geneva, 26-28 July 1989*. New York: United Nations, 1991.

A different problem is faced by psychiatrists who are asked to treat mental health problems of detained asylum seekers. Often such problems may be an appropriate reaction to the condition in which the person is held. For example, asylum seekers may have fled from oppression, leaving their family and possessions behind, only to be held indefinitely without charge. Psychiatrists asked to give treatment are in a difficult position, since the conditions under which asylum seekers are held are the very ones most likely to compound their problems. Medical treatment under these circumstances is unlikely to be totally successful.

Other abuses in which doctors can participate

The following affronts to human dignity were not considered in detail by the Working Party either because they did not apply to prisoners or because they represented a significant issue deserving of separate consideration.

Virginity testing

This practice — a particular form of intimate body search — was introduced in Britain in the late 1970s supposedly in order to verify statements made by young women arriving at British airports and claiming that they were the fiancees of British residents of Asian origin. The "test" was supposed to allow definitive determination of virginity, with an assumption that any found not to be virgins would not be betrothed and therefore bogus claimants of permission to enter the UK. After exposure in the press, the practice was halted by government order[63]. It is possible that virginity testing in some form or other continues as a cultural practice in various parts of the world though the Working Party had no evidence that it occurred as a result of government policy.

Forcible sterilization

The best documented example of this practice in recent times occurred in India under a policy implemented by the government of Mrs Indira Gandhi. In an attempt to encourage fertility control, the government at first offered rewards for men and women willing to undergo voluntary sterilization (though it might be argued that an inducement alters the

---

63 Phillips M, Dawson J. *Doctors Dilemmas*, pp.113-4.

nature of the consent to any given procedure) but later the formal necessity of consent was dispensed with and hundreds of woman (and men) were sterilized without their permission. This practice was halted in the wake of a storm of protest which followed the disclosure of the sterilization programme. In the People's Republic of China, the government has maintained a policy of one family-one child. This has led to considerable social pressures on parents to take aggressive measures to limit their family, including by contraception, abortion and sterilization[64]. A press report in August 1991 suggested that China was developing a programme to sterilise mentally retarded people who want to marry[65]. However, in both these cases, the Working Party felt the issues, though clearly having profound implications for medical ethics, were outside its remit.

Culturally-determined surgical procedures

In some cultures, certain surgical procedures are carried out on children in conformity with religious beliefs. These can involve different parts of the body, but the most controversial are those involving the male and female genitals. Male circumcision is rarely medically-indicated and female circumcision — better described as genital mutilation and ranging from removal of the hood of the clitoris at its mildest to complete removal of the clitoris and labia[66] — virtually never. The role of the doctor in carrying out such a procedure on children who cannot themselves consent thus becomes an important ethical issue. Reports that young girls were being circumcised in British surgeries in accordance with parental wishes prompted the introduction of legislation outlawing these practices[67]. This move was supported by the British Medical Association, which in 1983 passed a resolution supporting legislation against "female circumcision" except where a disease process is present.

---

64 A report on the *24 Hours* radio program [BBC World Service, 13 September 1991] presented allegations that pregnant women in one province of China were forcibly taken to clinics where their pregnancies were terminated.

65 China seeks to 'improve' population by sterilising the mentally retarded. *Guardian*, 17 August 1991.

66 The most severe form of female circumcision involves virtually the total excision of the external genitals and infibulation - the stitching together of the remnants leaving a small opening for micturition and passage of menstrual blood.

67 Prohibition of Female Circumcision Act 1985. In addition, s.47 of the Children Act 1989 gives local authorities investigative powers where there is reason to believe a child is likely to suffer significant harm as a result of female circumcision.

The Association also objects to training for cultural rites being given in the UK since this lends respectability to the procedures. Nevertheless, anecdotal evidence indicates a continuing interest in some sectors of the community in obtaining this procedure for social (i.e. non-therapeutic) reasons.

An active discussion has surfaced in connection with the role of the National Health Service in the provision of male circumcision in the light of serious sequelae to poorly carried out operations by technically unskilled religious "surgeons"[68]. Important as this issue is, circumcision is not imposed by government decision, nor is it practised on prisoners and it was felt therefore to be a phenomenon outside the Working Party's brief.

Experimentation on prisoners

The Declaration of Helsinki of the WMA sets out the standards for experimentation involving human beings and was a response to the experimentation carried out by the Nazi doctors during the second world war[69]. Prisoners have, in the past, been one of the vulnerable groups which participated in medical experiments of varying kinds. In 1906, 24 inmates of a Manila prison were experimentally inoculated with a cholera vaccine which, it transpired, was contaminated with the plague bacillus. None had given informed consent or authorization; 13 prisoners died. An investigative committee recommended an end to the exposure of a prisoner "to a dangerous or at least painful experiment against his will, without his consent clearly and freely given" which was, in any event, unlawful but the committee's conclusions appear to have been ignored[70].

However, such experimentation is not something only from the distant past and from the horrors of war. Reports of unethical medical experimentation continue to appear in the medical literature. A report of a United States House of Representatives subcommittee discussed in

---

68 Madden NP, Boddy S-AM. Should religious circumcisions be performed on the NHS? *British Medical Journal*, 1991; **302**:47. See also: Cohen J, Zoltie N. *BMJ*, 1991; **302**:788.

69 See: Mitscherlich A, Mielke F. *The Death Doctors*. London: Elek, 1961; Proctor R. *Racial Hygiene: Medicine Under the Nazis*. Cambridge: Harvard University Press, 1988. Less publicised were the horrific experiments carried out in Manchuria by Japanese doctors prior to, and during, the second world war. See: Williams P, Wallace D. *Unit 731*. London: Grafton, 1990.

70 Chernin E. Richard Pearson Strong and the iatrogenic plague disaster in Bilibid Prison, Manila, 1906. *Reviews of Infectious Diseases*, 1989; **11**:996-1004.

a leading article in the *British Medical Journal* revealed experiments such as the irradiation without consent of the testicles of over 100 prisoners in Washington and Oregon state prisons between 1963 and 1971 to determine a dose which would sterilize them[71]. Such experiments are totally unethical. The Working Party was not aware of any current experimental programmes in which consent was not sought or obtained and which were not for the benefit of the prisoner. However, it is concerned that considerable vigilance should be exercised over the possible abuses that could occur for whatever motives when researchers seek to involve prisoners in their studies.

Trade in human organs

Recent articles in the national and medical press have exposed a horrifying and totally unethical trade in human organs[72]. Such a trade caused deep concern to the Working Party and it was noted that it was in total conflict with the recently-promulgated WHO standards on organ transplantation[73]. Nevertheless, there was little evidence to suggest that governments themselves were coercing individuals to "donate" organs. Prisoners, especially those condemned to death, would be a particularly vulnerable "population at risk" of such abuses, and this issue warrants the close attention of those organizations monitoring prison situations. One case of concern already mentioned in chapter 6 is that of organ use from executed prisoners. Another is the use of reductions of sentences (or even amnesties) for prisoners who consent to give away a kidney[74]. Other aspects of the transplant trade ought not to be addressed under the rubric of government-directed torture and other politically-directed abuses involving doctors. The refusal of governments to adequately address the issue is, however, a major concern.

---

71 *American Nuclear Guinea Pigs: three decades of radiation experiments on US citizens*. Washington DC, Committee on Energy and Commerce, US House of Representatives, 1986. Cited in: Hamblin TJ. A shocking American report with lessons for all [editorial]. *British Medical Journal*, 1987; **295**:73.

72 Blood money. *Observer magazine*, 7 July 1991. Kandela P. India: kidney bazaar. *Lancet*, 1991; **337**:1534; Lam S-K. Kidney trading in Hong Kong. *Lancet*, 1991; **338**:453.

73 World Health Organization. Guiding principles on human organ transplantation. *Lancet*, 1991; **337**:1470-1.

74 Information from Johannes Wier Foundation, correspondence 17 January 1992.

Conclusion

The Working Party concluded that medical personnel did play a role in the involuntary feeding of hunger-strikers. It recognized that some doctors may do so as a result of deeply-held conscientious beliefs. Equally it recognized that some instances of forcible feeding were little short of torture and carried out under the orders of a government determined to impose its will on powerless individuals resorting to their only possible form of protest. We felt that feeding in the absence of consent is a procedure which should only be resorted to in exceptional circumstances: when the doctor is uncertain of the intention of the hunger striker; when the person refusing food is no longer competent to make a rational informed decision to fast; and when there have been significant changes in the circumstances which gave rise to the strike (for example, a change in government policy) and a prisoner is not able to give consent due to the effect of the hunger strike. Artificially feeding in such circumstances would seem to be compatible with medical ethics. However, if the intent is not to act in the best interests of the prisoner/patient, the doctor is likely to be in breach of established ethical principles. Further discussion of this issue is given in chapter 10.

We were equally persuaded that there is evidence that the denial of medical care to prisoner or detainees — often the result of a malevolent prison management policy — is sometimes due to decisions taken by doctors. This is inconsistent with basic medical ethics and efforts must be made to ensure such behaviour is exposed and eradicated.

The evidence that prisoners are forcibly medicated in the absence of medical indications was much more difficult to evaluate. There are certain undeniable facts - that psychotropic drugs are used in prisons, that they are used sometimes without the consent of the prisoner, that prisons (in Britain, and certainly elsewhere) contain numerous mentally ill prisoners who probably should be elsewhere, and that prisons contain some extremely difficult and antisocial prisoners. The difficulty comes in assessing whether prisoner X or prisoner Y really were mentally ill at the time they were forcibly given drugs; and if they were not mentally ill, whether the administration of the drugs was undertaken as an acute measure to avoid serious risk to the prisoner or to others. Were the drugs given "in good faith" or as a cynical exercise in control?

We were unable to make a judgment concerning the extent to which medication was used for unethical purposes of prisoner control. However, it seems to us that two separate measures could both address the fears of those who believe that drugs are being used for purposes of control and contribute to better health care practice within prisons. The first is to more clearly separate the medical and psychiatric services from the penal service. That is to say, the prisoner who requires medication would be referred for medical care in a medical facility where medical staff would have independence and control. (We recognize the difficulty posed by acute cases involving violence but believe that the clear separation of medical from penal functions could nevertheless contribute to diminishing this issue.) Furthermore, as the BMA has previously recommended in its 1990 *Working Party Report on the Health Care of Remand Prisoners*, prison hospital staff must remain as an exclusive resource to prison medical services and not as an additional resource to prison governors. The second measure is an appeal system similar to that already operating in many mental health care systems, including Britain's. The prisoner would be at liberty to try to prevent forcible medication and to appeal for evaluation of current medication. Some of these suggestions are embodied in the *Principles for the Protection of Persons with Mental Illness and for the Improvement of Mental Health Care* adopted by the General Assembly of the United Nations in December 1991[75].

The Working Party did not review any evidence which persuasively suggested that doctors had a major legitimate role in strip and intimate body searching. We recognize that it can be a humiliating experience and it is not without risk where the person to be searched does not consent or where the person carrying out the search is unskilled. However, we want to emphasise that doctors should only carry out such a search if requested by the individual concerned or, with their consent, where there are medical grounds for such a search. It is not the doctor's job to search for evidence to prosecute or help in management of prisoners on behalf of the police or prison authorities.

---

75 United Nations General Assembly Resolution 46/119; *op. cit.*

Chapter 8

Doctors as victims of repression: the need for international protection

In this century, and particularly since the second world war, the concept of the *neutrality* of the medical profession in conflict has been widely accepted. This neutrality was codified in the Additional Protocols of 1977 to the Geneva Conventions of 1949 at article 16[1]. In return for respect for neutrality, health personnel are expected to conform to certain principles, in particular to treat patients without regard to political beliefs, nationality or other factors. However, governments — and more particularly, military and security forces — differ widely in their respect for medical neutrality. Moreover, there are other contexts in which doctors and other health workers find themselves under attack. While considering the subject of medical involvement in human rights violations, it is important to understand the ways in which medical personnel become victims of abuses.

Doctors who take any stand against an unscrupulous government's human rights practices risk victimisation. We felt it important to illustrate the concrete problems faced by many colleagues in countries where human and professional rights are much more vulnerable than we are accustomed to. If we are to propose a stronger stand against pressure to infringe medical ethics then we must do so in the light of the real risk run by practitioners in different countries and circumstances. Many of the cases listed in this section have been the subject of BMA representations to governments and medical associations; examples of the actions which have been taken on behalf of persecuted doctors are given in Chapter 9.

---

1 International Committee of the Red Cross. *Commentary on the Additional Protocols of 8 June 1977 of the Geneva Conventions of August 12 1949.* Geneva: Martinus Nijhoff, 1987.

How doctors come to be targeted

A report by Amnesty International surveyed the victimization of doctors and other health personnel in the 1980s[2] and suggested that doctors can fall victims of repression because of their political activities, their defence of human rights, their professional activities (including criticisms of government policy or provision of health care to opposition figures), or as a result of a desire of a government to discourage opposition through terror or through making an example of well-known figures. In most circumstances reviewed by the Working Party, it was apparent that medical personnel were under attack for more than one reason. Thus, a doctor active in a human rights organization may well also have been politically active and have been, in his or her professional capacity, a critic of government policy. The context of repression summarized below is not intended to suggest that doctors live in a simple world of disconnected areas of social engagement but rather to illuminate some of the risks which dissenting doctors may face as a result of explicit or implicit government hostility.

While in most cases doctors are victimised by the state, on occasion they may be attacked by opposition groups. The reasons for this are varied: the most common reason being that by attacking health professionals, the population is deprived of health care. Over a period of time, the population will become demoralised and more susceptible to make concessions to the opposition. Recent examples of this occurred in Nicaragua and Mozambique.

Prosecution of opponents of psychiatric abuse: USSR

The first spate of books recounting personal stories of abuse by victims of Soviet psychiatric abuse were published in Europe and North America in the 1970s[3]. Throughout the 1970s, unofficial and hand-circulated reports — *samizdat* — further detailed extensive abuses of psychiatry for political purposes. In 1972, the Ukrainian psychiatrist, Semyon Gluzman[4], was arrested and charged under an article outlawing

---

2   Amnesty International. *Health personnel: victims of human rights violations.* AI Index: ACT 75/01/91, April 1991.

3   Medvedev Z, Medvedev R. *A Question of Madness.* London: Macmillan, 1971; Bukovsky V; *To Build a Castle.* London: Deutsch, 1978; Plyusch L. *History's Carnival.* London: Collins/Harvill, 1979.

4   This brief account is drawn from Bloch S, Reddaway P. *Russia's Political Hospitals.* London: Gollancz, 1977: chapter 8, *passim.*

anti-Soviet agitation or propaganda as a result of his reading and circulating *samizdat* material. His trial, from which his parents and friends were excluded, appeared to be based on the fact that he had given someone a copy of Alexander Solzhenitsyn's banned book *Cancer Ward*. It resulted in an astonishing seven-year sentence of imprisonment to be followed by three years' exile. It is widely believed that the real reason for his imprisonment was disputing the psychiatric diagnosis of the prominent military dissident, General Piotr Grigorenko.[5]

Grigorenko had urged democratization of Communist Party rules, including rotation of elected officers, for example. He was subsequently imprisoned for anti-Soviet activity. Following a short period in prison, General Grigorenko was found not legally responsible by psychiatrists from the Serbsky Institute (including Drs Morozov and Lunts) and was interned in a Special Psychiatric Hospital. He was again arrested in 1969 after four years of liberty and sent for psychiatric assessment to a Tashkent psychiatric commission which found him legally responsible for any actions he had taken. However, shortly thereafter he was flown to the Serbsky Institute where he was declared ill. The Serbsky commission found that:

Grigorenko is suffering from a mental illness in the form of a pathological (paranoid) development of the personality, with the presence of reformist ideas that have appeared in his personality, and with psychopathic features of the character and the first signs of cerebral arteriosclerosis.[6]

Dr Gluzman, and two colleagues whom he never identified, analyzed the reports of the two psychiatric commissions as well as Grigorenko's writings and asserted in a detailed 1971 commentary that the Serbsky doctors were either incompetent or had written deliberately false statements.

Dr Gluzman and his two colleagues concluded that General Grigorenko was:

not suffering from mental illness and his condition during the period of his activities to which the charges related cannot be considered a psychotic one of non-responsibility ... the decision of the [Serbsky]

---

5 For an account of Grigorenko's life, see: Reich W. The case of General Grigorenko: A second opinion. in: Stover E, Nightingale EO. *The Breaking of Bodies and Minds: Torture, Psychiatric Abuse and the Health Professions.* New York: Freeman, 1985.

6 *Ibid.* p.191.

commission that Grigorenko is mentally ill is not legitimate because it is not stated explicitly what changes in his personality gave grounds for equating his condition with mental illness.[7]

It is believed that this critique, made anonymously in a *samizdat* publication, was the root cause of Gluzman's harsh sentence. During his first few years of imprisonment he undertook several hunger strikes in protest against conditions in the prison. In 1974 he co-authored with Vladimir Bukovsky a *Manual on Psychiatry for Dissenters*. This resulted in further charges. Dr Gluzman was released at the end of his sentence in May 1982 and resumed work as a doctor (though not psychiatrist) in 1983[8]. He gave evidence to the BMA working party in June 1990, at which he described the harsh conditions, including forced feeding, to which he was subjected during his detention. He formed the independent Ukrainian Psychiatric Association at the beginning of 1991.

In January 1977 a small number of human rights activists in Moscow formed a Working Commission to Investigate the Use of Psychiatry for Political Purposes. By 1981, after publishing 24 *Information Bulletins* on psychiatric abuses, all members of the working Groups were either in prison or exile. The group comprised Alexander Podrabinek (5 years' internal exile), Irina Grivnina (5 years' internal exile), Dr Leonard Ternovsky (3 years in a labour camp), Vyacheslav Bakhmin (3 years' labour camp), Dr Alexander Voloshanovich (voluntary exile), Dr Anatoly Koryagin (8 years, imprisonment and labour camp, 4 years' internal exile). The two last-named were the psychiatric consultants to the commission[9]. Dr Koryagin was released in 1987 after having been subjected to extremely rigorous conditions of detention and having undertaken several hunger strikes. He now lives in exile.

Mass arrests in Syria

A state of emergency has been in place in Syria continuously since March 1963. It places all powers of internal and external security in the hands of a Martial Law Governor, in practice the Prime Minister, who delegates martial functions to the Minister of the Interior. These officials can order:

---

7   Cited in Bloch S, Reddaway P. *Russia's Political Hospitals*. London: Gollancz, p.115.

8   General Grigorenko was "rehabilitated" in 1991. See chapter 5.

9   Bloch S, Reddaway P. *Soviet Psychiatric Abuse: The Shadow over World Psychiatry*. London: Gollancz, 1984, pp.72-110 *passim*.

the placing of restrictions on freedom of individuals with respect to meetings, residence, travel and passage in specific places or at particular times. Preventive arrest of anyone suspected of endangering public security and order. Authorization to investigate persons and places. Delegation of any person to perform any of these tasks.[10]

Between 1978 and 1979, the Syrian Bar Association persistently urged reforms on the government, including an end to the state of emergency, guarantees of the independence of the judiciary, and protection of lawyers' freedom of expression. By January 1980, in the absence of any action by government, the General Assembly of the Damascus Bar resolved to call a strike for 31 January 1980 and called on other professions, including the medical association, to support it. On 31 January the head of the Bar Association held talks with government members and the strike was postponed. Joint meetings of medical, dentists, pharmacists, lawyers and other professional associations in March called for reforms. On 21 March 1980 the General Conference of the Syrian Medical Association passed a resolution asking for, *inter alia*:

- reaffirmation of the principle of the citizen's right to freedom of expression, thought and belief;
- denunciation of any kind of violence, terror, sabotage and armed demonstration, whatever the reasons and justifications;
- abolition of Exceptional Courts;
- release or trial of all detainees.[11]

On 31 March 1980, a national strike took place. A week later, a presidential decree was issued authorizing the dissolution of the councils of professional associations, and on the 9 April 1980, the entire structures of the medical and other professional associations were dissolved and in the following days numerous doctors, lawyers, engineers and other professionals were arrested.

In 1983, Amnesty International published a list of some 100 doctors, dentists and veterinarians who had been arrested in the wake of the

---

10 Article 4 of State of Emergency Law, Syria. Cited in *Report from Amnesty International to the Government of the Syrian Arab Republic*. London: AI Publications, 1983.

11 Amnesty International. *Chronological background and documents relating to the detention of members of the Syrian Medical, Engineers and Bar Association*. AI Index: MDE 24/08/83, 20 July 1983.

strike and dissolution of the professional associations[12]. In 1984 more information became available: the names of two of the arrested doctors who had been executed and several others who had been released reached Amnesty International from unofficial sources[13]. At no time has the Syrian government given any information on the fate of those who have now been held for more than a decade without charge or trial. As is detailed in chapter 9, the BMA has written numerous times to the Syrian government, the *Ordre des médecins syriens* (Syrian Medical Association) and the Association of Arab Doctors in Tunisia but has received no reply to these letters. While the suppression of the *Ordre des médecins syriens* at the time of the 1980 strikes probably represented the end of a free medical association in Syria, this increases our concerns rather than ameliorates them.

The Syrian Association is a member association of the World Medical Association, warmly welcomed into that body in 1981[14] and as such should be able to demonstrate a concern for the human rights and welfare of a significant number of doctors arrested and held without charge or trial for political reasons. Moreover, it should be able to find time to reply to letters of concern from a sister organization such as the BMA.

Civil unrest: El Salvador

In October 1979, a military coup brought a "reform" government to power in El Salvador. However, within months the civilians in the government withdrew leaving the military members in command. In January 1980 a mass protest in the capital San Salvador was attacked by army units, effectively ending peaceful public protest in that country. As the scale of violence increased, the political opposition was transformed into the illegal and revolutionary opposition. Widespread killings took place — between 9-10,000 in 1980 according to US government and Salvadoran human rights sources[15]. A commission to investigate attacks on health workers in 1980 noted:

---

12 Amnesty International. AI Index: MDE 24/07/83, 22 July 1983.

13 Amnesty International. *Further information on Syria: cases of doctors detained since 1980.* AI Index: MDE 24/04/84, 13 July 1984.

14 The Syrian Medical Association. *World Medical Journal*, 1982; **29**:11.

15 *Report on Human Rights in El Salvador.* Compiled by Americas Watch Committee and American Civil Liberties Union, January 26th, 1982. New York: Vintage, 1982, p.xxvi.

The brutality involved in the killings of health workers and patients and the accompanying torture suggest that this is a deliberate tactic aimed at striking terror into the hearts of others. Victims have been decapitated, emasculated or found with the initials 'EM' which stand for Esquadron de Muerte [Death Squad] in their flesh....

The risk of swift, brutal and fatal reprisal means that most health care professionals will necessarily have second thoughts about which patients they will treat.[16]

A further medical fact-finding mission to El Salvador in January 1983 sponsored by four US medical and scientific organizations[17] in cooperation with the International League for Human Rights investigated the fate of 16 health professionals reported to have disappeared in 1982 as well as examining other health-related issues in El Salvador. Their report[18] continued the unrelenting bad news from that country: Dr Manuel de Paz, secretary general of the trade union of the Salvadoran Social Security Institute, disappeared on 28 January 1982; Carlos Vargas, professor of physiology at the National University of El Salvador, disappeared on 16 December 1981; René Vazquez, oncologist and former secretary general of the trade union of the Salvadoran Social Security Institute, disappeared on 19 January 1982. While in El Salvador, many further cases were brought to their attention: Juana Cisneros, a 47-year-old nurse abducted while waiting for a bus in front of her hospital and whose whereabouts were unknown; Juan Garzona, 45-year-old surgeon shot to death in front of his house; Romeo Gonzalez, a hospital doctor abducted by armed men from his house and later found dead with evidence of an explosion on his abdomen. Further reports in the period since then suggest that medical personnel continue to be at risk in El Salvador as a result of the civil conflict and the poor human rights record of the Salvadoran military[19]. Many of these

---

16 *Abuses of medical neutrality*. Report of the Public Health Commission to El Salvador, July 1980. Committee for Health Rights in El Salvador. New York, 1980, p.4.

17 The organizations were the American Association for the Advancement of Science, the Institute of Medicine of the National Academy of Sciences, the National Academy of Sciences and the New York Academy of Sciences.

18 *Report of a medical fact-finding mission to El Salvador, 11-15 January 1983*. Washington: American Association for the Advancement of Science, April 1983. 16pp.

19 See Eisenberg C. et al. Health and human rights in El Salvador. *New England Journal of Medicine*, 1983, **308**:1028-9; San Francisco Committee for Health Rights in El Salvador. *El Salvador 1985: Health, Human Rights, and the War*. A report of the third US Public Health Commission on El Salvador.

casualties reflect the lack of respect for the neutrality of medical personnel during a conflict[20].

After a period of steady decline in political killings, there was an upsurge in 1988. In June 1989, the US organization Physicians for Human Rights (PHR) sent a delegation to El Salvador to investigate violations of medical neutrality and other abuses of human rights reportedly carried out by both sides in the conflict and in November 1989 one PHR delegate returned to determine what had happened during the upsurge in the conflict which occurred in late 1989. The PHR investigation found that medical neutrality was not respected by the Salvadoran authorities, that both the government and the armed opposition (FMLN: *Frente Farabundo Martí de Liberación Nacional*) failed to identify adequately medical personnel and hospitals and impeded health care delivery, and that the Salvadoran military had "attacked, tortured and, in some cases, killed medical personnel and patients"[21].

In the following year a report by the US-based International Commission on Medical Neutrality recorded that the "arrest or detention of 28 health promoters, 6 medical students, 5 first-aid or ambulance workers, 5 physicians, 2 nurses, 17 otherwise undescribed hospital workers, and 1 dental technician were reported [by human rights monitors during the period November 1989 to November 1990]". The report commented that "there is evidence to suggest that in most cases health workers are arrested or detained as punishment for carrying out their medical duties", a finding consistent with earlier observations[22].

Attack on human rights organization: Chile

The most prominent doctor to become a casualty of the military coup in Chile in 1973 was the president, Dr Salvador Allende. In the immediate post-coup period, a number of doctors and students disappeared following arrest by military agents[23]. Despite persistent efforts to determine the fate of these individuals, no information has been

---

20 Examples are given in Amnesty International. *Health personnel: victims of human rights violations*. *Op. cit.*

21 Physicians for Human Rights. *El Salvador: Health Care under Siege: Violations of Medical Neutrality during the Civil Conflict*. Somerville: PHR, 1990, p.72.

22 *Violations of Medical Neutrality: El Salvador*. A Report by the International Commission on Medical Neutrality. Seattle: ICMN, March 1991, pp.16-17.

23 Amnesty International. *"Disappearances" of medical professionals in Chile*. AI Index: 22/100/83, January 1984.

forthcoming. In subsequent years several doctors active in human rights and politics were arrested and imprisoned or banished. In 1986, a doctor working with the Catholic human rights organization, the *Vicaría de la Solidaridad*, was arrested together with other colleagues, as a result of his role in providing medical care to an injured man who claimed he had been hit by a stray bullet during a confrontation between police and armed opposition in Santiago. The man, Hugo Gomez, sought help from the *Vicaría*. He was examined by Dr Ramiro Olivares who thought the man's story to be credible — injuries to bystanders due to street confrontations involving police and armed opposition were common at the time — and referred him to a private clinic after opening a normal medical file for him. In fact, the man had been a participant in the confrontation and some days after his initial medical assessment four staff from the private clinic were arrested followed later by the arrest of Dr Olivares and a *Vicaría* lawyer, Gustavo Villalobos. One doctor was released but the rest were charged under the Arms Control Law. The *Colegio Médico de Chile* publicly supported the doctors on the grounds that doctors should provide medical care without political consideration.

In late May and early June 1986 two more doctors were arrested, though by August 1986 all of the doctors had been released on bail. In December 1986, the charges against Dr Olivares and three others were changed to the more serious anti-terrorist law offenses. On 12 December 1986, Dr Olivares entered prison where he remained for one-and-a-half years. On the pretext of investigating the incident, the government tried to get access to all the *Vicaría*'s medical records though this was resisted — successfully — by the organization. In June 1990, the charges against Dr Olivares were revoked at a Supreme Court hearing, three months after the end of military rule. Other doctors in the case who were still under prosecution eventually also had their cases dropped or reviewed by the incoming government of Patricio Aylwin.

Arrest of health workers during mass demonstrations: China

The increasing protests in favour of democracy in China during 1989 culminated in the "occupation" of Tiananmen Square by thousands of students during May and early June 1989. On the night of 3/4 June 1989, the People's Army entered the Square and put an end to the protest. Among the thousands of students, academics and workers arrested following the crackdown, the cases of five health workers have come to light. Two, Dr Song Song, a surgeon, and Dr Shan Gangzhi, a urologist, were volunteers on medical duty in Tiananmen Square during the night of the military action. Both were arrested during June 1989 and their whereabouts are not known. The three others, Dr Wang Xuezhi of the College of Chinese Traditional Medicine in Beijing, Zhao Yiqiang, a research technician from Beijing Medical University, and Liu Feng, a 19-year-old second year student of public health, were arrested in June and August 1989 and little is known of their fate[24]. Other prisoners held since the Tiananmen Square arrests are known to be in poor conditions and in August 1991 two of those with long prison sentences began hunger strikes.

Criticism of government health policy: Vietnam

Dr Nguyen Dan Que, a 50-year-old endocrinologist, has spent many years imprisoned in Vietnam for political reasons. After graduating in medicine at Saigon University and a period on the medical school teaching staff, he undertook WHO-sponsored studies in Paris, Brussels and London (where he studied at the Royal Postgraduate Medical School, Hammersmith Hospital). He returned to Saigon from London in 1974 where, in 1975, he was appointed Director of Cho-ray Hospital. He was soon making criticisms of the public health policy of the new government which had come to power following the defeat of the South Vietnamese forces in April 1975. As a result of his critique, he was dismissed from his post and in February 1978 was arrested and accused of "rebelling against the regime". He was imprisoned without charge or trial for a ten-year period.

In February 1988 he was released. He subsequently became a founder member of the Humanist Movement, a non-violent political opposition movement. In May 1990, the Movement launched a petition calling for political change in Vietnam including the introduction of a multi-party system of government. On 14 June 1990, Dr Nguyen was re-arrested. He was subsequently charged under Article 73 of the Criminal Code with "activities aimed at overthrowing the people's government".

On 29 November 1991 he was convicted and sentenced by the People's Court of Ho Chi Minh City to 20 years' imprisonment and five years' house arrest[25].

---

24 Physicians for Human Rights. *Medical Action Alert: China*. Somerville: PHR, 31 July 1991.

25 Amnesty International. *Viet Nam. Nguyen Dan Que: prisoner of conscience sentenced to 20 years*. AI Index: ASA 41/02/92, January 1992.

Sudden change in government by coup: Sudan

On 30 June 1989, the civilian government of Prime Minister Sadiq al-Mahdi was ousted in a military coup which brought General Omer al Bashir to power. All political parties, associations and trade unions were banned including the Sudan Doctors' Union and other professional associations. In November 1989, the Sudan Doctors' Union called a seven-day strike in protest at the political situation and in support of a memorandum which it had submitted to the government. Dozens of doctors were arrested, many of whom were beaten and later released. Some doctors were subjected to torture. Four of those detained were tried in December 1989 with holding a ten-minute meeting to declare the strike. Two of those charged were acquitted but Dr Maamun Mohamed Hussein was convicted of "calling and organizing a strike" and "incitement to opposition against the government" and was sentenced to death. The other doctor, Sayed Mohamed Abdallah, was sentenced to 15 years' imprisonment. The sentences provoked international outrage and in May 1990 both doctors were released, shortly before a two-member delegation from the American Association for the Advancement of Science was due to arrive in Khartoum to investigate the human rights situation. In August 1990, however, Dr Abdallah was again arrested and held for several months without charge.

In April 1990 Dr Ali Fadul, who had lost his job following the doctors' strike, was tortured to death. His body was taken to a military hospital in the early hours of 22 April by members of the security services. According to a report in the *Lancet*, two army doctors performed a necropsy and gave the cause of death as cerebral malaria. An independent opinion suggested that the cause of death was cerebral trauma. He was buried secretly by the security police and his family was not permitted to attend the burial. No proper investigation was held and no credible explanation of his fate has been given by the government[26]. In mid-1991, some 20 health personnel were still in prison without charge or trial.

There have been persistent reports since the 1989 coup that conditions for prisoners are appalling with inadequate food, non-existent or primitive health care, poor hygiene and extremely harsh conditions. The human rights organization Africa Watch reported in February 1991

---

26 Anonymous. Sudan: repression of doctors. *Lancet*, 1990; **336**:1307.

numerous cases of prisoners in need of medical care[27]. One prisoner held at Shalla prison, 500 km from Khartoum, suffered serious complications of a compound fracture of the femur. The fracture occurred during a trip to Khartoum following his arrest. He was admitted to Gedaref hospital but did not receive adequate treatment for five days. He was then transferred to Obdurman military hospital and then to Shalla prison. Because of the delays in his treatment, doctors later recommended that he would require an amputation.

The provision of adequate medical care was not necessarily appreciated by the authorities. Some of the doctors working at el-Fasher hospital, the nearest hospital to Shalla, were reputed to provide excellent medical care to prisoners and as a consequence of this were removed from their posts in May 1990[28].

Doctors victimised for humanitarian actions: Turkey

In March 1991 the BMA appealed to the Turkish authorities for the release of Dr Cemal Kahraman, President of the Human Rights Association in Nusaybin, Turkey. He was detained on his return from a visit to Omerli, for which he had gained permission, to collect the bodies of five guerrillas of the Kurdish Workers Party who were shot in a clash near the town. Dr Kahraman was charged on 12 April 1991 and committed to prison. It appears also that Dr Kahraman was subjected to torture during detention in police custody.

It later emerged that, as a result of his humanitarian actions, in which he collected the bodies of five guerrillas of the Kurdish Workers' Party (PKK) to return them to their families, Dr Kahraman was charged with membership of the illegal PKK. He stated during the hearing that he had been tortured during this detention, including being subjected to a mock execution and being suspended by his arms with his wrists tied behind his back. He was further subjected to psychological torture which included threats to rape his wife and being made to witness other prisoners being tortured.

It is reported that although Dr Kahraman bore marks of torture his injuries were not documented during the medical examination. He has made a formal complaint to the Chief Prosecutor and asked that legal

---

27 *News from Africa Watch.* Sudan: Inside al Bashir's prisons. Torture, denial of medical attention and poor conditions. 11 February 1991. 20pp.

28 *Ibid.*, p.5.

action be taken against the torturers but no investigation has yet been opened.

In another torture case, Dr Hüseyin Özkahraman, a representative for the Kadiköy district of Istanbul of a national community movement[29], was arrested on 6 July 1991. He and other members of the organization had gathered in front of their premises to issue a press statement opposing the closure of their branch. He was interrogated by two police officers who beat him, after which he had difficulty breathing and swallowing. They attempted to force him to sign prepared statements, but he refused to do so. After being released by the Kadiköy State Prosecutor he asked to be sent to a Forensic Medical Institute (FMI) and he was subsequently sent to Cerrahpasa FMI from where he was referred to Haydarpaşa Numune Hospital. There it was noted that he had sustained a perforated eardrum, and had marks of blows to one eyebrow, face and various parts of his body. Kadiköy FMI certified that he was unfit to work for 15 days. A case was opened against a police officer but it was dismissed when Dr Özkahraman was unable to identify the officer. The case was referred back to the Kadiköy State Prosecutor.

Invasion: Kuwait

The invasion of Kuwait by military forces of Iraq on 2 August 1990 ushered in a period of apparently unrestrained human rights violations characterised by gross brutality. Hospitals and medical personnel were not accorded any special rights and a number of doctors suffered the same fate as hundreds of other Kuwaiti citizens and residents. Iraqi troops entered hospitals in Kuwait City in the weeks that followed the invasion, looting equipment and harassing staff. Information was very difficult to obtain as the country was occupied by a particularly brutal force and those fleeing gave what, in some cases, later turned out to be inaccurate but highly dramatic information about killings by Iraqi troops. Nevertheless, reports from Amnesty International[30], Physicians for Human Rights[31] and Middle East Watch[32] all agree that hospitals

---

29 The Halkevleri (literally "people's houses") is a community-based social movement carrying out cultural, educational, advisory and solidarity activities. It is not affiliated to any political party.

30 Amnesty International. *Iraq/Occupied Kuwait: Human rights violations since 2 August [1990]*. AI Index: MDE 14/16/90, 19 December 1990, 82pp.

31 *Iraqi-occupied Kuwait: the health care situation*. A report by Physicians for Human Rights/Denmark and Physicians for Human Rights/USA, March 1991, 35pp; Human Rights (UK). *Kuwait 1991: Human rights abuses and effects on the health*

were attacked by Iraqi troops and that health workers were harassed, arrested, tortured or killed in the period following the invasion. For example, an obstetrician named variously as Hisham al-'Ubaidan, Hahisham al-Obaidan or Hisham Obaidan[33], who worked at the al-Sabah Maternity Hospital, was killed in early October 1989 outside his home. The reason given in two of the reports was the treatment he gave to members of the Kuwaiti resistance. He was reported to have been tortured before his killing. All the reports record other examples of attacks on hospital personnel, and threats and actual injury or death to other health workers.

Ethnic conflict: Yugoslavia

Yugoslavia has seen increasing ethnic tensions within the different constituent republics which has reached a tragic climax in the civil war which started in 1991. In the Serbian autonomous region of Kosovo there has been widespread discrimination against ethnic Albanians, which led to the mass dismissal of Albanian surgeons, doctors and other health workers[34]. The medical school was virtually closed to Albanian students; medical care for the Albanian population was said to be put at risk. The BMA communicated with the authorities and the Yugoslav Medical Association in response to telefaxed appeals from Albanian doctors but was unable to obtain any response.

In another republic, on 25 June 1991, Croatia declared its independence from the Yugoslav federation. This was fiercely contested by the Serbian republic and the Yugoslav National Army (JNA). The army intervened in the name of protection of the Serbian minority in Croatia and the maintenance of the Yugoslav state. In the ensuing conflict, about one-third of Croatia's territory fell to JNA forces and Serbian paramilitaries. Atrocities and massacres were alleged on both sides. The town of Vukovar in Croatia was besieged and the hospital, sheltering some 1,000 patients, was shelled for 86 days. At the fall of Vukovar, on 20 November 1991, the acting head of the hospital,

care system during and after the Iraqi occupation. Undated [1991].

32 Middle East Watch. *Kuwait: Deteriorating human rights conditions since the early occupation.* November 1990.

33 The transliteration of Arabic names into English gives rise to a variety of versions according to the conventions used. The first version comes from the AI report, the second from the PHR (Denmark/US) report and the third from the PHR (UK) report.

34 Dobreci S. Yugoslavia: repression of doctors in Kosova. *Lancet*, 1991; **338**:302.

Dr Vesna Bosanac, was arrested and imprisoned in Sremska Mitrovica prison in Serbia. On 23 November, Radio Belgrade broadcast allegations about her and another Croatian doctor, referring to Dr Bosanac as "alias Mengele" and implicating her in the fate of 93 mutilated bodies outside the hospital and the murder of 15 children nearby. Along with many other organizations, the BMA issued a series of urgent appeals. Dr Bosanac came to BMA House on her release shortly afterwards to describe her experiences and to urge appeals for an end to the conflict. To the extent that it can be judged at this time, it appears that doctors on both sides have acted in the spirit of medical ethics in their treatment of both combatants and non-combatants. No doubt a clearer picture will emerge in due course.

Killings by opposition movements

Sometimes doctors and other health personnel are victimised by opposition movements. In Nicaragua, for example, during the period of the civil war of the 1980s, local health workers were among targets of the armed opposition, the so-called *contras*.

> By December 1987, a total of 48 health workers, including 25 doctors and 9 nurses, had been killed by *Contras*.... Another 32 had been kidnapped and 26 wounded. Some of those kidnapped, including Dr. Gustavo Sequiera, Vice-Dean of the Managua Medical School, and Dr Myrna Cunningham, now Governor of Northern Zelaya Province, were high-ranking medical leaders. Most victims, however, were young nurses and doctors working in isolated rural communities.
>
> In some cases, health workers were targeted and murdered while carrying out their professional duties. Such an attack claimed the lives of nurse Juana Cruz Padilla and ambulance driver Ambrosio Raudales Lopez, on 28 March 1983, as they were taking a patient by ambulance to Ocotal hospital. Both were tortured before being killed.[35]

A doctor in charge of a *Contra* medical organization was quoted in a US magazine explaining the reason for health worker casualties:

> The *brigadistas* [voluntary health workers] are working with the enemy. They are a legitimate target. These people should not be in the war zones. The Sandinistas are using them for propaganda....[36]

---

35 Garfield R, Williams G. *Health and Revolution: the Nicaraguan Experience.* Oxford: Oxfam, 1989, p.68.

36 Cited in *ibid.*, p.69.

Mozambique was also the victim of a prolonged civil war waged by an opposition force (Renamo: *Resistencia nacional Moçambicano*), supported first by Rhodesia and later by South Africa. By 1977 its objectives were formulated: to "sabotage, to disrupt the population and to disrupt the economy"[37]. As part of this strategy, health clinics were targeted.

> By the end of 1985, 196 peripheral health posts and health centres had been destroyed and another 288 had been looted and/or forced to close....Official Ministry of Health statistics list 15 kidnapped workers but in Zambezia province alone more that 30 health workers were kidnapped in 1985.[38]

In both the above cases the reasons for opposition attacks on health workers appeared to include a policy of demoralization of the population in areas under the control of the government, for the simple practical reason that health clinics are a "soft target", as well as for reasons of creating general terror and intimidation of professionals and intellectuals.

The need for international protection

As with all human rights abuses, the most basic step in defence of those affected is to expose the existence of the abuses and let the government involved know that they are not going unnoticed[39]. Human rights organizations such as Amnesty International report that some governments are very sensitive to their image and will take steps to investigate and redress allegations of torture and other violations. Other professionally-based organizations such as Physicians for Human Rights also report signs of sensitivity on the part of offending governments. Of course, there are governments which are less sensitive to public exposure, though this is not an argument in favour of remaining silent, and publicity serves other important functions. Most important is that the detainee or prisoner can learn of the interventions being made on his or her behalf through family, friends or lawyers. At a wider level,

---

37 Vines A. *Renamo: Terrorism in Mozambique.* York: Centre for Southern Africa Studies, University of York, 1991, 176pp. [quote from p.16]

38 Cliff J, Noormahomed AR. Health as a target: South Africa's destabilization of Mozambique. *Social Science and Medicine*, 1989, **27**:717-22.

39 Wiseberg LS. Protecting human rights activists and NGOs: what more can be done? *Human Rights Quarterly*, 1991; **13**:525-44.

outside support offers solidarity with domestic human rights activists. The experience of the BMA is that action by the Association is warmly appreciated by sister associations and individuals under threat.

Article 6 of the Declaration of Tokyo suggests that doctors who oppose human rights violations through their adherence to the Declaration should receive the support of the World Medical Association which will also encourage the support of the international community. No formal mechanism exists to express such support though the WMA has regularly written in support of detained doctors and on one occasion undertook a mission to Chile following the detention of the President and Secretary-General of the *Colegio Médico de Chile*[40]. It appears to the Working Party to be unacceptable for the medical profession to express a resolute opposition to human rights violations and to medical involvement therein without at the same time making a commitment to support actively those doctors who courageously live up to their ethical principles and are persecuted for doing so.

There is an apparent absence of any systematic international support of the medical profession generally, and individual practitioners in particular, at risk of human rights violations. The World Health Organization does not have, for example, a committee equivalent to the International Labour Organization's Committee for Freedom of Association which works to ensure the free functioning of trade unions' and employers' associations. Both the World Medical Association and World Psychiatric Association (WPA) have taken individual *ad hoc* actions in support of individuals though there is no systematic and visible mechanism for addressing the problem. Some of the activities of the WMA have been mentioned above. The WPA has made some protestations towards the Soviet government regarding individual psychiatrists under threat and has conferred an honorary membership on one particular psychiatrist, Anatoly Koryagin, in recognition of his role in opposing Soviet psychiatric abuse. However, the activities undertaken by the WPA are a minor contribution compared to the efforts made by national bodies and non-governmental organizations. It is not clear whether this reflects the nature of the WPA secretariat which has no permanent staff, or whether it is a result of a policy decision to adopt a very cautious approach to involvement in appeals on human rights issues.

---

40 Wynen A. Report: WMA mission to Chile. *Danish Medical Bulletin*, 1987; **34**:192-3.

Finally, there is an argument for renewing efforts for ensuring that codes of medical ethics adequately address the issues of obligation on the doctor but also that those who uphold the codes of ethics will receive the full support of the profession at an international level. This would require more than passing all the responsibility for action on to the shoulders of the World Medical Association but rather an active commitment on the part of national bodies to support any colleagues who are in serious need of moral and practical help.

Chapter 9

The response of the medical profession

Just as it is not possible to document every individual act of unethical behaviour by a doctor in the face of human rights violations, so it is equally difficult to document fully each positive and sometimes heroic affirmation of law and medical ethics in the face of attempted violations of human rights. However, if we are to make a concrete attempt to increase the effectiveness of ethical codes it is important to assess the extent to which medical personnel can and do assert their principles and conscience in difficult circumstances and at personal risk.

Resistance to medical involvement

Unarguably, formidable pressures can be brought to bear on doctors to assist in dubious if not openly illegal or unethical procedures. Where the doctor's life is at risk or where threats have been made or implied against the safety of the doctor's family, it is understandable that there might be a feeling that there is no choice but to comply. Examples of this were given in chapter 4. However, there is also evidence available which shows that doctors can refuse to cooperate in torture and can document its effects. Sometimes it is a question of courage which appears to be beyond the average. The documentation provided by doctors in countries as diverse as Chile and the former Soviet Union, in the face of persistent intimidation, is an example. In other circumstances, it seems more a question of personal will and political and professional support; it is this last which appears to us to be crucial in the fight to keep doctors out of torture chambers, and the role of medical associations is particularly crucial.

Medical Associations: the track record

Not unexpectedly, the picture is uneven with respect to the role of medical associations in the defence of human rights. Indeed, it is only relatively recently that such a role has been formally discussed by medical associations[1]. In Latin America, medical associations responded to human rights violations in different ways at different times. This was in part explained by the fact that they were controlled for certain periods by the military governments which held power in their countries, though some associations were dominated by doctors sympathetic to the government of the day and unmoved by human rights violations, even those practised against doctors[2]. Moreover, the structure of the organizations of medical professionals varied in different countries, resulting in the possibility of conflict between different parts of the medical profession. In Chile, for example, the national *Colegio Médico* is the principal body representing doctors' interests in professional and ethical matters and was able to make pronouncements on ethical issues at national level, whereas in Brazil, by contrast, there are Medical Councils (*Conselhos Médicos*) at state and federal level governing the ethics of the profession, Medical Associations (*Associacãos médicas*) which deal with scientific aspects of medicine, and the Medical syndicates (*Sindicatos médicos*) which negotiate with the authorities on behalf of doctors, creating the potential for state and federal bodies to pull in different directions.

It is invidious to single out associations for particular praise or criticism. However, mention should be made of some professional associations for the steps they have taken to reduce medical involvement in human rights abuses. Several of the medical bodies discussed below changed policy as a result of changes in the nature of the military governments under which they worked. The Brazilian *Conselho Médico de São Paulo* investigated allegations that a forensic doctor, Harry Shibata, had falsely certified that the politician Marco Coelho had no signs of physical abuse following a period of detention and torture by the security police, the DOI-CODI. The *Conselho* took several years to reach a determination because in the period between the complaint to the Council (1976) and the voting in of a new Council Executive (1979) no significant effort was made to address the issue. The new executive

---

1　See Coloquio Internacional. *Rol de las Asociaciones Médicas en la defensa de los Derechos Humanos.* [28,29 November 1985.] Santiago: Colegio Médico de Chile, [1986]. The meeting was subjected to police harassment despite its professional focus and the presence of international participants.

2　See the account of the debate within the Colegio Médico de Chile immediately prior to and after the military coup of September 1973. Hamilton G. Professionalism — Lessons from Chile [parts 1 and 2]. *Medicine and Society*, 1982; 7(2,3):14-17 and 7(4):30-33.

commenced investigations which led in 1980 to a decision to assess the charges and to arrive at a decision. Dr Shibata was struck off but the decision was reversed on appeal to the Federal Council. Although, therefore, he was technically still able to continue his medical career, in fact he did not work again in forensic medicine.

In Chile, the *Colegio Médico* spent a decade after the 1973 military coup, deprived of the right to elect its own officers. The *Colegio* was bitterly divided at the time of the coup and in the immediate post-coup period appeared to side with the incoming military government. However, by the time the government restored the right of the organization to elect its own officers, there was a strong mood for reform and for self-criticism of the record of the association.

> From 1973 to 1981 ... the leadership of the Chilean Medical Association was insensitive to reports of violations of human rights brought to its attention by physicians and other Chilean citizens. These violations included killings, 'disappearances', and academic dismissals. It is painful to recognize that the CMA was a mere spectator to the institutionalized violence taking place around it. The association failed to protest this violence, inquire about its causes, and denounce those responsible. Moreover, the association disclaimed reports that physicians were present during the torture or ill-treatment of detainees held in centers run by the security forces.[3]

The association immediately launched a vigorous campaign to promote a wider knowledge of international standards such as the Declaration of Tokyo (which it paid to have published in a Santiago daily newspaper[4]) and to work on its own ethical code. As a result of its internal discussions, the ethical code of the Chilean association deals with the subject of medical involvement in torture in some detail and with subtlety. The code of ethics which arose from these considerations contained clear instructions to doctors seeing prisoners, including in provision 1:

> The doctor may never attend any person under the following conditions:
>   If the doctor is prevented from identifying himself.

---

3   Minutes, General Council of the *Colegio Médico de Chile*, Santiago, 1 November 1985; cited in Stover E. *The Open Secret: Torture and the Medical Profession in Chile*. Washington: American Association for the Advancement of Science, 1987, p.47.

4   *El Mercurio*, 27 November 1983. Cited in: Amnesty International. *Human Rights in Chile: the Role of the Medical Profession*. AI Index: AMR 22/36/86, September 1986.

If the doctor is covered or hooded, or his identity is in any other way concealed.
If the patient is blindfold (for non-medical reasons) or in any other way prevented from seeing the doctor.
In any place of detention other that his home or a publicly recognized place of detention.
In the presence of third parties who impede free contact or alter the normal relationship between doctor and patient.[5]

The association also investigated persistent allegations that medical personnel were directly implicated in the torture of people detained by the security forces. At the time of writing 12 cases have been investigated and six doctors have been found culpable of participation in human rights violations and have been subjected to penalties ranging from reprimand to expulsion[6]. An enquiry about the behaviour of a thirteenth doctor opened in March 1991 and is still in progress, though the fate of the inquiry is uncertain following the departure of the accused doctor from Chile[7].

In Uruguay, the two medical associations — the *Sindicato Médico* (based in the capital, Montevideo) and the *Federación Médica del Interior* (representing provincial doctors) — had leadership imposed by the military in 1975[8] and remained under military control for several years. In 1984, in the last months of the military government, the Seventh Medical Convention erupted when one of the doctors present made allegations about the involvement of another Convention participant in human rights violations. This provoked a heated debate[9] which could not be resolved at the meeting but which did give impetus to the establishment of a national commission of medical ethics to investigate medical involvement in human rights violations during the

---

5   From *Ethical Principles Relative to the Medical Care of Detainees*. Santiago: Colegio Medico de Chile, 1985. The ethical guidelines also require any doctor compelled to breach any of the Association's standards to report the fact within five working days.

6   Stover E. *The Open Secret... op. cit.*; Rivas F. *Traición a Hipocrates: Médicos en el Aparato Represivo de al Dictadura*. Santiago: CESOC, 1990.

7   Dr Gunter Seelman, Human Rights Department, Colegio Médico de Chile: interview, Santiago, 27 November 1991.

8   Goldstein R, Gellhorn A. *Human Rights and the Medical Profession in Uruguay since 1972*. Washington DC: American Association for the Advancement of Science, 1982.

9   Si, me referia a Ud. [Yes, I am referring to you]. *Jacque* [Montevideo], 27 July 1984.

military period. The tribunal held investigations into allegations against some 80 doctors and eventually expelled five from the medical associations after finding them culpable of acts incompatible with medical ethics[10].

In addition, the medical associations have actively promoted the independence of doctors working within the military and have maintained links with overseas associations with the common concern for the role of medical ethics in protecting both doctor and patient from abuses such as torture.

The response from the *Conferación Médica de la República Argentina* (Argentine Medical Confederation) has been more ambiguous. There have been no publicly reported investigations into the behaviour of doctors during the "dirty war" (1976-83) nor public exposure of medical assistance in torture. Even Dr Berges, a doctor notorious for taking part in torture sessions, who was convicted in a court of law and sentenced to six years' imprisonment in December 1986, was apparently not formally disciplined by the national association at the time[11]. Nor has the Confederación responded to several letters sent to its General Secretary by the BMA Working Party, regarding allegations about Argentinean doctors. However, at the 1983 Assembly of the World Medical Association, the Argentine Medical Confederation representative combined with the Chilean Medical Association representatives to co-sponsor a draft resolution reiterating the substance of the Declaration of Tokyo[12].

In the absence of a clear lead from the organized medical profession, a number of doctors established an unofficial commission against impunity to publicise the role of doctors in torture. Some of the members of the commission were subjected to threats and, in one case, a car bombing.

On the negative side, the failure of the All-Union Scientific Society of Psychiatrists and Narcologists to protest or take any other steps to

---

10 See Martirena G. *Uruguay: la tortura y los médicos*. Montevideo: Ediciones de la Banda Oriental, 1988.

11 He was however expelled by his local medical association, apparently to return to practise elsewhere.

12 The draft resolution was not accepted by the meeting on procedural grounds as it had not been submitted in advance to the resolutions committee. The key clauses of the draft motion were to express protest at attacks on physicians, to condemn participation of physicians in torture and ill-treatment of prisoners and to support member national associations which were enforcing ethical standards and investigating cases of alleged abuses involving physicians.

address the widespread abuse of psychiatry in the USSR for at least two decades, represents one of the most demonstrable failures of a professional association to address a serious and systematic abuse of medical expertise (see chapter 5). Letters to the Society from the BMA about alleged ethical abuses failed to elicit any response.

Likewise, attempts by the BMA to raise human rights issues with the medical association of Syria have met with a total lack of response over a period of several years. Given that the subject of much of this correspondence was the fate of some 100 doctors, most presumed to be association members, held without charge or trial in various prisons in Syria, this lack of response is particularly regrettable.

The apparent disinterest of the medical association in the fate of colleagues suggests that the association supports the doctors' imprisonment or is under such restriction by the government that it regards any protest as too dangerous. Given the fate of the doctors detained during 1980 in Syria, and the measures taken against the Syrian Medical Association at that time, either of these possibilities may in fact be the case. The Syrian Medical Association is a member of the World Medical Association, joining the year following the mass arrests referred to above.

The Turkish Medical Association has attempted to give guidance to its membership on ethical issues as well as to investigate allegations of medical breaches of ethics. In 1985 six members of the executive committee of the TMA wrote to the government urging the abolition of the death penalty. They particularly wanted doctors to be relieved of what they saw as an unethical role in executions. The executive committee members were subsequently charged with an offence under the Law of Associations which prohibits political statements by associations. They were later acquitted after a long trial.

In the following year the association drafted a code of ethics which specified in article 16 a prohibition on any involvement in torture and presence at an execution[13].

A sign that change is possible in the practices of a medical association is given by recent developments in the practices and policies of the Medical Association of South Africa (MASA). The Association was seriously discredited in the late 1970s by its total failure to address adequately the subservience to the police of district surgeons attending Steve Biko, the black consciousness leader who was fatally injured by

---

13 Amnesty International. *Turkey: Torture and medical neglect of prisoners*. AI Index: EUR 44/28/88, May 1988, p.10.

police beatings in 1977[14]. This failure and the World Medical Association's acceptance of MASA back into the world body led in part to the BMA's withdrawal from the WMA in 1984.

In the decade following the Biko affair, there were continuing allegations that South African district surgeons failed to act with clinical independence and to fulfil any protective role towards prisoners, many of whom were held under the Internal Security Act without any legal redress[15]. The magnitude of this failure was underscored by the action of one district surgeon, Dr Wendy Orr, who sought court protection for prisoners under her responsibility when she found evidence that they were being ill-treated by police and prison personnel. Her intervention remains the only case of a district surgeon seeking legal remedies through the courts to protect prisoners[16].

The South African regulatory body, the South African Medical and Dental Council, appears not to have found anything to cause ethical problems to doctors in South African prisons in "the practices of torture, detention without trial, solitary confinement or *apartheid medicine*"[17]. The SAMDC appears not to have made any public statement on any of these subjects, nor to have given guidance to South African doctors as to what to do when their ethical principles conflict with the orders of the State. The SAMDC position on torture is that it "supports the Tokyo Declaration"[18].

In the recent past there have been signs that MASA is changing, undoubtedly due, in part, to the pressure put on the association by South African human rights and health groups and adverse international publicity and criticism. The depth of this change is difficult to determine but there has been a flurry of declarations on human rights themes. A recent positive development has been the drafting of guidelines on the

14 Silove D. Doctors and the state: lessons from the Biko case. *Social Science and Medicine*, 1990; **30**:417-29.

15 Rayner M. *Turning a blind eye? Medical accountability and the Prevention of Torture in South Africa.* Washington: AAAS, 1987.

16 Dr Orr's action was not without a price - "after the Supreme Court action she was prevented from seeing detainees and reassigned to other medical duties. She also received telephoned death threats." *Apartheid Medicine: Health and Human Rights in South Africa.* Report of a AAAS medical mission of Inquiry to South Africa in April 1989. Washington: American Association for the Advancement of Science, 1990, p.79.

17 *Ibid.* pp.94-5.

18 *Ibid.*, p.95.

handling of hunger strikes which represents the first cooperative undertaking between MASA and NAMDA (see chapter 7).

There remains, however, a lack of clarity about the instructions which MASA is prepared to give to doctors working for the state, i.e. district surgeons, and about what disciplinary measures it is prepared to implement in order to defend principles embodied in the Declaration of Tokyo. With impending changes within South African medicine, reforms in this direction are on the agenda.

BMA activities

As a result of decisions taken in the 1960s, the BMA has an active practice of contacting medical associations about apparent violations against medical personnel abroad or where there are credible allegations that doctors are involved in serious abuses of medical ethics and human rights. The BMA regards this practice as part of the commitment to the WMA's Declaration of Tokyo which promises in article 6:

> to support the doctor and his or her family in the face of threats or reprisals resulting from a refusal to condone the use of torture or other forms of cruel, inhuman or degrading treatment.

The BMA has taken action in many of the cases detailed in this and the previous chapter. For example, in addition to writing numerous letters to the Syrian Medical Association and the Union of Arab Doctors based in Tunis on behalf of Syrian colleagues detained since the strike, the BMA contacted diplomatic representatives in Damascus in an attempt to gain further information. On the same issue, it has also lobbied the European Parliament, whose President has raised the BMA's concerns on several occasions.

On behalf of doctors detained in Sudan, including Dr Maamun Mohamed Hussein, Dr Sayed Mohamed Abdallah and Dr Ali Fadul, the BMA has sent letters and telegrams, and issued a press release to the UK press in an attempt to raise awareness about the situation. The procedure which the BMA observes in taking action on cases forms appendix 1. A summary of the BMA's activities and of the results of its inquiries are given annually in the BMA Council report which is included as a supplement to the *British Medical Journal*.

In addition to writing letters, the BMA has taken an active role in several important initiatives. For example, it has taken part in international meetings on medical and human rights themes. In 1985 it was represented at the International Colloquium convened by the

Colegio Médico de Chile by the Secretary, Dr John Havard[19]. In 1989 Dr John Dawson, as head of the Association's Professional, Scientific and International Affairs Division, participated in a meeting organized by the French medical commission of Amnesty International in Paris on the theme of 'Medicine at Risk: the doctor as human rights violator or victim'. Some of the recommendations of that meeting reflected the input made by Dr Dawson[20].

The following year he contributed to an international symposium on 'Torture and the Medical Profession' which was held in Tromsø, Norway, in 1990[21]. His successor, Dr Fleur Fisher, contributed to the follow-up conference in Budapest in 1991. One development of the Tromsø meeting has been a proposal for the establishment of an International Tribunal for the Investigation of Torture, which is mentioned below. Perhaps the most significant contribution of the BMA to the prevention of torture was the publication in 1986 of its first report on the subject: *The Torture Report*.

The World Health Organization

The WHO is sensitive to political forces. The threat of the withdrawal of US funding to the WHO if the organization admitted the Palestine Liberation Organization as a full member is a recent example of this[22]. Thus, while it has undertaken some extremely successful public health initiatives, including the abolition of smallpox, it has had a peculiarly eclectic position on human rights. It has played a major role in documenting the health effects of apartheid for example[23], and more recently has undertaken a program on AIDS which included a strong

---

19 Havard JDJ. Doctors and Torture [editorial]. *British Medical Journal*, 1986; **292**:76-7.

20 See Recommendations of Working Party 3, in *Doctors and Torture*, London: Bellew, 1991, pp.142-4.

21 The papers from this conference were published as a supplement to the *Journal of Medical Ethics*, December 1991; **17** (4).

22 The application for WHO membership by the Palestine Liberation Organization on 14 April 1989 was based on the PLO's declaration of Palestinian statehood made in December 1988. The US Secretary of State, on 1 May 1989, threatened to recommend withdrawal of all US funding to any organization admitting the PLO. Consideration of the application was subsequently postponed to the 1990 meeting where it was defeated. *Keesing's Record of World Events*, 1989, **35**:36672, and 1990, **36**:37474.

23 *Apartheid and Health*. Geneva: WHO, 1983.

human rights component[24]. It introduced the UN Principles of Medical Ethics which were adopted by the General Assembly of the UN in 1982. However, it has not addressed issues such as the protection of doctors under persecution for respecting the UN Principles nor the question of the response to doctors convicted of assisting the practice of torture. It is not unrealistic to expect that the major inter-governmental health body should address these issues.

International Associations

The World Medical Association and the World Psychiatric Association as well as numerous more specialized international organizations represent the professional and ethical interests of doctors at an international level though their representativeness is patchy. The World Medical Association, of which the BMA was a founding member in the immediate post-war period, has suffered something of a crisis in its identity in the period after the Tokyo Assembly in 1975. Formed with the active participation of the BMA in 1947, the WMA was seen as an important international response to the egregious abuses of medical ethics to which doctors were a party during the 1939-1945 war. One of its first actions was to draft a code of international medical ethics and, in its more than 40 years of existence, it has continued to debate ethical issues and to formulate principles for the guidance of national associations.

However, from its inception its intended universality was eroded by the Cold War and the North-South divide. Further problems arose when tensions about South Africa developed within the WMA membership. In 1977, the killing of the South African "black consciousness" leader, Steve Biko, precipitated another crisis when, following the dismal failure of MASA to address adequately the failure of Biko's doctors to protect their patient, MASA was welcomed back into the WMA. This led to the withdrawal of all black African medical associations (with the exception of the anomalous Medical Association of Transkei — see below) and contributed to the withdrawal of the BMA which, like some other European associations, was also unhappy about the voting system which applied within the WMA. The European "dissidents" together with the Canadian Medical Association and some other non-members formed a loose network known as the "Toronto group"; discussions

---

24 *Report of an International Consultation on AIDS and Human Rights; Geneva, 26-28 July, 1989.* New York: United Nations, 1991.

within this network canvassed the idea of establishing an alternative international body but this was rejected and instead discussions with the WMA for re-entry of members of the Toronto group were initiated. In 1985 the Uruguayan member association withdrew over what it saw as WMA reluctance to adopt a strong enough stand on human rights.

In the past few years there have been signs that the representativeness of the WMA is assuming a more truly international nature: a medical association from the People's Republic of China joined (prompting a change in the Taiwanese association's name from the Chinese Medical Association to the CMA Taipei) and associations from the former USSR, other Eastern European associations and north Africa were admitted. In 1991, a number of associations formerly affiliated to the Toronto group rejoined the WMA though the BMA decided to remain outside the Association for the present time.

There remain idiosyncrasies in WMA membership. In some countries the national representative is not the main medical association (the WMA is not well-adapted to deal with the fact that some countries have several medical associations with none being agreed as the national representative organization); for one country the member association does not represent that country's doctors[25]; and one recently-withdrawn "national" member association did not represent a recognized state[26].

In a letter to the Working Party in October 1991, Dr André Wynen, the Secretary General, explained the limitations on how the WMA promulgates its codes and disciplines breaches of them. He made clear that the WMA is always willing to undertake appeals on behalf of threatened doctors and gave examples of some WMA successes. He said that, with regard to ensuring compliance with the Declaration of Tokyo, there was no mechanism for giving it teeth[27].

The World Psychiatric Association has its own running sore — the issue of Soviet psychiatric abuse — on which it has attempted to rub a mild salve. Its activities on other human rights aspects of psychiatry have been even milder. The issue of Soviet psychiatric abuse has been dealt

---

25 There is no member association representing doctors working in Cuba. There is, however, a Miami-based organization representing exiled Cubans and Cuban-American physicians — the *Colegio Médico Cubano Libre* (the Free Cuba Medical Association).

26 The Transkei Medical Association comes from a South African homeland which is recognised only by South Africa and (implicitly) by the World Medical Association. It was removed from WMA membership against its wishes in 1991.

27 Letter to Working Party, October 1991.

with briefly in this report. The WPA was split by arguments between those who saw criticism of the Soviet member association as representing an unwelcome intrusion of politics into a professional arena, and those who saw the issue as completely within the remit of a professional debate. And of course the cool breezes of the Cold War blew round the debaters. Despite the efforts of reformers, the Committee established in 1977 to investigate individual cases of political abuse of psychiatry has not made any significant findings.

The WPA has not visibly taken up cases of detained psychiatrists (though it may have done so on a confidential basis) and has not been prolific in adopting positions on ethical and human rights issues. Exceptions have been a summary of WPA comments on the Human Rights Commission draft Principles for the protection of persons with mental illness[28] and a statement on psychiatric involvement in the death penalty[29]. This relatively low profile on human rights and ethics may reflect the lack of resources of the WPA secretariat, which transfers to the office of the incoming Secretary-General after each sesquiennial Congress or it may have to do with a deliberate policy not to get involved with the hot issue of human rights in the wake of the bruising issue of Soviet psychiatric abuse.

By contrast, the International Council of Nurses has taken quite strong stands on human rights issues likely to pose challenges to nurses. For example, it has adopted several statements on nurses and human rights and has tended to take a stronger line than the medical associations. For example, where the WMA and the WPA have opposed medical involvement in capital punishment, the ICN has urged member nursing associations to argue for its abolition[30].

The Commonwealth Medical Association has been involved in contributing the Commonwealth Human Rights Initiative[31] but has not adopted any policy of active intervention in individual cases. This is a significant gap as human rights issues arise regularly in many Commonwealth countries.

---

28 WPA Statement and Viewpoints on the Rights and Legal Safeguards of the Mentally Ill (adopted by the WPA General Assembly in Athens, 17th Oct. 1989). *WPA Bulletin*, 1990; **1**:29-33.

29 For text of the 1989 declaration see the appendices.

30 International Council of Nurses. *Position Statement on the Death Penalty and Participation by Nurses in Executions*. Adopted, Seoul, 1989.

31 Commonwealth Human Rights Initiative. *Setting the World to Rights: Towards a Commonwealth Human Rights Policy*. London: CHRI, 1991.

In short, there is considerable potential for international associations to take more positive steps both to support individual practitioners and member associations when they face pressure to participate in, or overlook, abuses and to promote more effective observance of international ethical standards.

The role of other non-governmental organizations

A number of non-governmental organizations (NGOs) exist expressly to campaign on human rights issues, some with particular reference to medical themes. For example there are organizations which campaign generally on human rights such as Amnesty International (AI) and Human Rights Watch, plus numerous national organizations. Other organizations focus specifically on torture. These include the Association of Christians for the Abolition of Torture and SOS-Torture. On specifically medical and human rights issues there are AI medical groups in 30 countries; branches of Physicians for Human Rights in the UK, US and Denmark; the Dutch Johannes Wier Foundation; and many others bodies in both developed and developing countries which are actively pursuing aspects of the rights of citizens to access to health care and freedom from human rights violations[32]. There are also organizations such as Médecins sans Frontières, Médecins du Monde and others which contribute directly to giving deprived populations access to primary health care and numerous bodies providing special care to victims of human rights violations. In several countries, centres which offer medical treatment for torture victims have been set up, and perform valuable work in documenting cases of torture as well as campaigning vigorously against it. These centres include the Medical Foundation for Care of Victims of Torture in London, the establishment of which was commended in the BMA's first report on torture and which has since grown in size and in achievement.

The International Council of Health Professionals (ICHP), which was intended by its progenitors to be a sister organization to the International Commission of Jurists, has recently been wound up. This will leave a gap which is (or could be) partially filled by the WMA. The particular value of a body such as the ICHP is that it can look at ethics without

---

32 We did not actively seek to survey the groups around the world working in this field. Thus the groups noted here are those known through publications or correspondence. We are aware of the existence of many such groups, including in countries where human rights violations are a daily reality. They have our admiration.

regard to the sensitivities of national associations which will, of necessity, have a national view reflecting a certain degree of self-interest.

The International Committee of the Red Cross holds a particular place in the international medical sphere. While it does not campaign publicly on medical and human rights issues beyond urging observance of the Geneva Conventions, it plays a vital role in reviewing the application of humanitarian law. The ICRC visits prisoners of war, as stipulated in the Third Geneva Convention of 1949. It also visits prisoners not specifically protected by international humanitarian law. In this case, the ICRC strives to prevent forced disappearances, to eradicate torture and to improve conditions of detention. ICRC doctors play a key role in these activities[33].

These diverse organizations offer a useful reminder to the medical profession of the expectations held by society of the positive role which doctors and professional associations can play. They have organized meetings, published books, undertaken missions, promoted ethical and professional standards, contributed to the work of the United Nations and generally stimulated medical associations to involve themselves in defending ethical standards in the face of governments which wish to subvert national and international law.

Proposal for an International Tribunal for the Investigation of Torture

Proposed by the Montevideo group[34], the Tribunal aims to investigate and judge "crimes against humanity, especially torture and other maltreatment" for which members of the medical or legal profession are alleged to be responsible. In March 1991, the Tribunal statutes were drafted and nominations for membership invited[35].

At the time of writing, it has yet to be formally constituted and its status and relations with other legal bodies are unclear.

---

33 Reyes H, Russbach R. The role of the doctor in ICRC visits to prisoners. *International Review of the Red Cross*, No. 284, 1991.

34 The Montevideo group comprises the Medical Associations of Uruguay and Denmark, and the Rehabilitation Centre for Torture Victims in Copenhagen.

35 Esperson O. Statutes for the International Tribunal for Investigation of Torture. *Journal of Medical Ethics*, 1991; **17**, Supplement:64.

The impossible dilemma — hero or victim

Can we insist that the doctor never assists in the commission of an abuse whatever the circumstances? Can we insist that the doctor be prepared to sacrifice his or her life in defence of the individual or even of medical ethics in the abstract? We do not think so. We are not heroes and don't feel it proper to insist that all other professionals should be. Undoubtedly there are some doctors whose resistance to abuses has been extraordinarily brave and inspirational. Some of these have been detailed above. However, we must address the central issue which was well summed up in a Council of Europe document:

> The intolerable choice between complicity and heroism — between the side of the torturers and that of the victims — should not be left to the individual conscience. It is incumbent on all of us, on each national and supranational community, to elaborate rules and conventions, but above all *concrete* rules, which not only prohibit participation in torture but effectively protect the doctor against the risks to which refusal to assist torture will expose him or her.[36]

What appears clear is that the individual doctor surrounded by men with guns is in a very weak position to assert moral beliefs let alone put them into practice. For this reason the Working Party believes that it is vitally important that some effort is made to prevent doctors from being placed in impossible positions and to alleviate as much as possible the individual doctor from having to make agonizing moral decisions while under duress. This means several things must be done. The standards of medical ethics must be clearly disseminated among doctors and must be made known to government and government agencies. The medical association must play a leading role in setting and monitoring standards and, crucially, the association and other relevant bodies must commit themselves to the support of those who uphold the standards which the association is proclaiming.

The medical profession must be seen by the individual doctor as a natural ally and source of advice and support. Where doctors are coerced into deviating from their code of ethics they should be able to report this to the association in the expectation that the association will

---

36 Lore C, di Georgi S, Pogliano C. La torture. In: Proceedings of a Council of Europe Colloquium: *Le médecin et les droits de l'homme*, March 1982. Strasbourg: Council of Europe, 1985, p.155. Cited in Amnesty International. *Involvement of medical personnel in abuses against detainees and prisoners.*

deal with the infraction with understanding and compassion and with a determination to persuade the government that such coercion is unacceptable. Drawing a line between unacceptable capitulation and dangerous risk-taking is not easy and we have tried to suggest a way forward in our recommendations at the end of this report.

Chapter 10

Monitoring the threat

What are the signs of the slide towards systematic human rights abuse? The answer to this question is usually most easily provided in retrospect. With the benefit of hindsight, the slow or rapid breakdown of the rule of law can often be analyzed step by step. However analyzing the current state of human rights at any given moment is often made difficult by the political dimension of the subject and the extent to which we regard our own society as "normal" and deserving support. In order to try to address this problem, the Working Party has given particular thought in this chapter to areas where we see potential erosion of rights in the United Kingdom.

There are some aspects of the free society whose progressive loss should ring alarm bells to those concerned with preservation of human rights. This report focuses on the medical role in defending (or failing to defend) human rights. However, medicine is practised in a political framework and there are a number of political "indicators" which point to a fragile state of human rights and medical ethics. Each in itself is not necessary for torture or unfailingly indicative of the existence of torture. Rather they point to a situation where the abuse of human rights can more easily occur or be covered up.

The key elements in the protection of human rights have been referred to in several analyses[1] and what follows draws on these and other sources. While these have a perspective wider than the practice of medicine, it is indisputable that any significant loss of democratic rights will have implications for medical professionals.

Declared respect for international standards

Human rights standards are just words — at least they remain just words if they are not put into practice. Governments can, if they are serious,

---

1   Amnesty International. *Torture in the Eighties*. London: AI, pp.77-89; Stover E, Nightingale EO. *The Breaking of Bodies and Minds*. *Op. cit.*; AI Medical Commission, Marange V. *Doctors and Torture*. London: Bellew, 1991.

give clear signals that they intend to protect human rights. The following questions give a clue to government intent:

- Has the government ratified international human rights instruments? Failure to take this fundamental step is a bad omen.
- Has the government translated international human rights standards into domestic law? Are the international standards reflected in professional Codes of Practice?
- Are there domestic laws which transgress international standards? In many cases, emergency powers risk compromising human rights. Emergency legislation permitting detention without trial and similar measures may be brought in as a temporary move but kept in place for many years. The Syrian government declared a state of emergency in 1963. It is still in place. Administrative detention, widely practised in the Israeli Occupied Territories, has allowed for prolonged detention of Palestinian prisoners without trial. Administrative procedures can often be renewed without adequate possibilities of challenge.

The Official Secrets Act, which was introduced in response to a crisis but which cannot be regarded currently as emergency legislation, remains in force in amended form in British law. Prior to amendment in 1989, it had major implications for doctors working in government institutions as was illustrated in the case of one doctor in Northern Ireland who apparently resigned in the face of the gag imposed by the Act at a time when allegations of beatings in police custody were rife[2]. While not presenting a direct threat to the integrity of the population, it was widely regarded as a barrier to free speech by doctors and others in government institutions. Some argued that the Act permitted suspect practices and inferior standards to persist. The revised Act has yet to be tested in court.

The UK Prevention of Terrorism Act is another piece of legislation characterised by speedy introduction and long life. It was introduced as a rapid response to IRA terrorism in the 1970s and has been renewed annually ever since. It allows for detention without charge for seven days in contravention of international standards[3].

---

2 See Phillips M, Dawson J. *Doctors' Dilemmas. Op. cit.* p.108.

3 The European Court of Human Rights ruled in the case of *Brogan and Others* (29 November 1988) that the Act was in breach of the European Convention on Human Rights. This led the government to declare on 14 November 1989 that it would derogate indefinitely from Article 5(3) of the Convention which specifies, in

The judiciary

The way in which the judiciary operates is also indicative of the state of human rights in a country:

- Are judges independent? Is there an adequate appeals procedure to challenge legal decisions? Is there an effective complaints machinery? In some countries the deterioration in the human rights situation has been marked by the failure of the judiciary to assert their rights and responsibilities; in others there *is* no judicial independence and no rights of defence or appeal.
- Do trials conform to accepted international standards? Do defendants have access to independent lawyers? Is financial help such as "legal aid" available? Breaches of standards particularly likely to lead to abuses of human rights are mass trials and lack of an adequate appeals procedure.
- Are there identifiable groups in society which are treated differently by the police or judiciary? In Britain, blacks are more highly represented in prisons than whites on a per capita basis; on death row in the USA the same phenomenon is observable.

In the United Kingdom in 1991, the government attempted to remove legal aid from asylum seekers. A number of recent controversial cases have concerned the expulsion of people from Sri Lanka and Zaire. In November 1991, the European Court of Human Rights heard the case of *Vilvarajah and Others v United Kingdom* which involved five Sri Lankans who had been forcibly returned to their country, where a number of them were subsequently alleged to have been detained and ill-treated[4]. Britain was held not to be in breach of the European Convention, partly on the grounds that "ill-treatment must attain a minimum level of severity" and although "there existed the possibility that they might be detained and ill-treated, as appeared to have occurred in previous cases, a mere possibility of ill-treatment was not in itself sufficient to give rise to a breach of Article 3"[5]. Such a judgement may not seem satisfactory in that it would appear the individual, wishing to make a case for asylum, must almost be able to guarantee that any ill-

---

effect, that detainees should be promptly charged or released following arrest.

4 The first, second and third applicants claimed that they were arrested and detained and, save the first, ill-treated by members of the Indian peace-keeping force. The fourth claimed he was arrested and beaten by the police.

5 *Times* Law Report, 12 November 1991.

treatment meted out on his return will exceed the minimum level permitted in Europe.

Police stations

In many countries, prisoners may be detained and tortured in police cells rather than in prisons. The point of maltreatment in such cases may be to obtain a confession. Some of the same points that we would raise in relation to prison practice are therefore relevant to police detention.

- Does the detainee have a right to see a lawyer or doctor upon request?
- Are interrogation sessions tape-recorded, video-taped or subject to monitoring?
- Are uncorroborated confessions accepted as sufficient for a conviction?

In the UK, there has been evidence coming to light over the past few years of gross miscarriages of justice due in part to flaws in police practices and lack of protective measures for those accused. In some cases there were political overtones to the cases; in others not. In any event, it was noticeable that the victims were, in the main, members of minority groups.

Prison practice

Torture and similar abuses of human rights violations occur most commonly following arrest or abduction. The holding of prisoners without contact with the outside world is a practice which facilitates torture and other abuses. Therefore, in looking at a country's penal practices, we should ask:

- Are prisoners informed of their rights at the time of arrest and imprisonment? Is incommunicado detention permitted? Do prisoners have the right to visits by lawyers, doctors, families? Are prisons and other places of detention open to regular inspection?
- How are vulnerable groups such as women and children treated in detention? Is the detention of children permitted? Are female prisoners given adequate protections; are they questioned always in the presence of female guards? Are they given access to their children and family? Is strip searching practised? With what protections?

- Are prisons visited by independent observers? Is the investigating authority separated from the imprisoning authority? Do prisoners have to sign documents waiving rights or verifying good treatment? Is there a clear chain of command within the detaining or interrogating authority? It is important for the judicial system to ensure that investigation is carried out in the most impartial and accountable manner possible.
- Do prisons keep detailed records? Are they available to the prisoner's lawyer? Records become crucial when allegations of ill-treatment are made or when a prisoner dies in detention, and offer protection for both the prison authorities and prisoners.
- Are deaths in custody automatically investigated? Are they investigated by personnel outside the prison service? Are findings made public?[6]

The Working Party is very aware that doctors working in isolated situations in this country, particularly those employed by organizations such as the prison service or the Armed Forces, which are not primarily concerned with health and may be coercive, may be most at risk of becoming involved in suspect practices. We took note of Amnesty International's presentation of evidence to the UN in October 1991 about alleged maltreatment of suspects at Castlereagh holding centre in Belfast. In this case, doctors are not implicated in maltreatment but rather it is doctors who have drawn attention to the complaints of brutality.

Prisons in the United Kingdom were severely criticized in 1991 in a series of reports by both the Chief Inspector of Prisons, Judge Stephen Tumim, and the European Committee for the Prevention of Torture and Inhuman or Degrading Treatment[7]. Although it is a positive sign that such reports are published, the Working Party is concerned by the delays sometimes involved. In the case of Judge Tumim's report on Wormwood Scrubs, his account of "depressing and unsatisfactory conditions" was only published in December 1991, more than a year

---

6 For investigation standards and forensic protocols see *Manual on the Effective Prevention and Investigation of Extra-Legal, Arbitrary and Summary Executions*. New York: United Nations, 1991.

7 *Report of the European Committee for the Prevention of Torture and Inhuman or Degrading Treatment or Punishment (CPT) on its visit to the United Kingdom from 29 July 1990 to 10 August 1990*. CPT/Inf (91) 15. Strasbourg: Council of Europe, 26 November 1991. (The reply of the British Government is given in CPT/Inf (91) 16, published together with the above.)

after he inspected the jail. This is of concern to the BMA, whose membership includes doctors working in such prisons. Prison conditions affect not only the detained inmates but also the staff and it may be of little comfort for them to read Judge Tumim's verdict that "organization of medical services was seriously inadequate, with little staff training in AIDS and no organized health education. Defects were made tolerable only by a sensitive, sensible staff."[8]

Medical practice in prisons

The role of the doctor in a prison should be solely to provide medical care for inmates. It is not the doctor's role to assist in prison discipline or management. Therefore the issue of the independence of the medical service from the prison service is of great significance.

- Do prison doctors have, or act with, clinical independence? In Libertad Prison in Uruguay, information given by prisoners to prison doctors was systematically given to prison personnel in order to assist in controlling the prison population. In this report, we have shown that doctors working in the prison system may see their primary responsibility as being to the authorities, rather than to their patients. Do prisoners have access to their own, or at least an independent, doctor? The prisoner is a vulnerable person. Where there is a problem between the prison doctor and the prisoner, access to a second, preferably independent, doctor can overcome this problem.
- Are forensic and clinical activities kept entirely separate? Where a prisoner is interviewed or examined for forensic purposes when the prisoner is under the impression that what he or she says is protected by confidentiality, then there is a risk of compromising basic medical ethics and encroaching on fundamental rights of the accused or the prisoner.
- Is medical treatment given coercively? In what circumstances? What options are available to the prisoner to appeal against forcible treatment? Are experiments carried out on prisoners? If they are, what safeguards are in place?
- Is the identity of the patient known to the doctor and vice-versa? Many ex-prisoners who have been tortured report that they were kept blindfolded during medical examinations. Concealment of the identity of a patient must raise suspicions in the mind of the doctor.

---

8 Quoted in *The Guardian*, 19 December 1991.

- When an injured prisoner is brought for treatment, is there a plausible explanation for the injury? Are doctors asked to prescribe treatment without seeing the patient. In the Averroes hospital in Morocco (chapter 7), doctors prescribed medicines for prisoners held in the hospital basement without having seen them.
- Is there a medical association which acts independently? It is not insignificant that in several countries under dictatorship, such as Sudan and Syria, independent associations, including medical associations, are repressed or have imposed on them government-appointed leaders. It is the task of the medical association to maintain a distance between the profession and the state.

Mental health facilities

The Working Party noted the existence in England of two external inspectorates for the sphere of mental health treatment. We felt that the Mental Health Act Commission, although limited in the type of case in which it may formally intervene, has access to informally observe conditions on a wider scale. Unacceptable standards in psychiatric hospitals led the government to also establish the Health Advisory Service. We regret the apparent diminution of the powers of the latter, which no longer initiates visits but has to be invited by the Health Authority to carry out an inspection. The limitation in HAS powers is particularly disturbing, as current policies to provide care in the community lead to psychiatric units becoming progressively more isolated and increasingly run by non-medical managers.

Conclusion

Doctors can contribute to the preservation of democratic freedoms, not only by maintaining ethical and human rights standards but, through their professional associations, by keeping a watchful eye on the state. The relationship between the state and the doctor can at times be uneasy and there is often a conflict between the interests of the doctor and those of the government, particularly where the government wishes to involve doctors in aiding the political or security objectives of the state. It is the task of the medical association to maintain a healthy distance between the profession and the political apparatus while remaining responsive to medical and health issues of importance to the public and the government.

Chapter 11

Conclusions and recommendations

The Working Party commenced its deliberations with the knowledge that a number of organizations had published evidence of medical involvement in torture, among them the United Nations (UN Special Rapporteur on Torture), Amnesty International, the American Association for the Advancement of Science, and the British Medical Association itself which concluded its 1986 report by stating that:

> We have been shocked by incontrovertible evidence of doctors' involvement in planning and assisting in torture, not only under duress, but also voluntarily as an exercise of the doctor's free will[1].

The evidence available to the present Working Party reinforces this conclusion. We have received convincing evidence that even within the period since the Working Party was established, doctors have actively assisted in the carrying out of torture by others. We have also seen examples of unethical behaviour by doctors and other health personnel, as well as activities which caused us a certain amount of disquiet even if they could not be definitively regarded as unethical.

We found that doctors had actively participated in the process of torture by certifying the prisoner's fitness for torture, reviving the prisoner after collapse, monitoring the prisoner's state during torture and giving false or inadequate medical care to the tortured prisoner. Equally importantly, we found that many doctors who know that torture or other abuses are happening do nothing to challenge it. While acknowledging that in some circumstances this will require some bravery, the widespread failure to do *anything* about it suggests that there is a continuing need for the medical profession to restate that tolerating abuses is inconsistent with medical practice.

---

1 *Torture Report*, p.28.

A common form of collaboration in human rights abuses — sometimes intentional, sometimes not — is the writing of inadequate medical certificates for both living and dead victims of human rights violations. In some cases, the certificates are blatantly false and are intended to protect abusers and to obstruct the legal process. As this weakens the chances of the victim or his or her family obtaining recompense and justice, it again is totally in conflict with ethical, as well as humane, standards of behaviour.

The abuse of psychiatry as a substitute for embarrassing political imprisonment appears to be lessening. No new cases were found by a delegation of the World Psychiatric Association delegation which visited the USSR in mid-1991, though it found that the process of change was extremely sluggish and there was a failure to address the need for rehabilitation of former victims. In other countries the level of alleged abuse of this type is limited and can be expected to decrease in the future as democratic processes are strengthened and independent professional associations are formed. However, continuing vigilance is clearly needed and critical discussion of the relationship between psychiatry and the state should continue.

Hunger strikes are a common form of action undertaken by detained people to focus attention on their protest. The response of the prison authorities to such initiatives varies considerably as does the response of the medical profession. At its worst, the treatment of hunger-strikers is tantamount to torture as the powerless prisoner is kept chained and dirty and fed forcibly by nasogastric tube. In other circumstances, the prison authorities talk with the hunger-striker and permit medical personnel to manage the prisoner, as they would any other patient, in accordance with the ethical standards they hold. The role of the doctor in a hunger strike is clear where the clearly-expressed intent of the prisoner is known but is more complex in the absence of such knowledge, as will be evident in our recommendations below.

We found evidence that doctors play a role in the carrying out of corporal punishments and executions in several countries. Doctors examined prisoners to determine fitness or competence for the punishment and were present during the carrying out of the punishment: to prevent death on the one hand and to ensure death on the other. Doctors also have assisted in the development, and sometimes in the carrying out, of such penalties. The Working Party opposed the role of the doctor in the carrying out of corporal or capital punishments as contrary to medical ethics. We also found other aspects of medical involvement unacceptable. Thus, advising or training non-medical staff to carry out such punishments seemed unacceptable to us, because we believe that doctors should not contribute to the carrying out of punishments.

We support the position of the World Medical Association, expressed in the 1981 resolution on capital punishment, that the only role for a doctor at an execution is to certify death, but believe that there is a need to assert more vigorously what is not ethically acceptable. One such unacceptable role, in our view, is standing by the soon-to-expire prisoner giving advice to the executioner. Death can be certified away from the site of execution. Those acts (for example the preparation of lethal injections) which contribute more or less directly to the death of the prisoner appear to us also to be outside an ethical medical relationship with prisoners. We noted with extreme concern the proposals, now being implemented in some countries, to use the organs of executed prisoners for transplantation purposes. While transplantation surgery is a wholly worthy thing, the use of organs from prisoners whose capacity to freely consent must be in grave doubt seems to us extremely undesirable. The potential conflict of interest between the prisoner's legal rights to appeal and seek clemency and the possible need for his or her organs seems a real and unhealthy one.

With regard to corporal punishment, we discussed the role of both medical ethics and cultural values in its importance in any given society. It is likely that in all societies there are some people who would like to see corporal punishment retained or introduced as a disciplinary measure[2]. While we were opposed to the use of corporal punishment, whether whipping or amputation, fundamentally we addressed the ethical issue: should doctors participate? We felt not. It is not the role of the doctor, in our view, to assist the state to inflict punishments. Moreover, we could see no adequate medical method of protecting the prisoner from harm merely by visual inspection during the whipping (and of course it is a total nonsense to suggest a protective role for a doctor at an amputation unless one is to talk of "good" and "bad" amputations).

While religious values must be acknowledged and taken account of — and in this context, particularly Islam — it is striking that only a minority of Islamic countries practise corporal punishment (which in any event is not one of the five pillars of Islam). The Working Party took

---

2 In the United Kingdom, for example, support for corporal punishment is periodically expressed in the House of Commons by a small number of members of parliament. (See, for example, p.86 above.)

note of the humanizing aspects of Islam and felt that the progressive limitation of corporal punishment within the Islamic world reflected this.

The issue of forcible medication of prisoners, while simple to evaluate in principle, was a very difficult one for the Working Party to assess in practice. This was partially due to the lack of information available and, more importantly, the difficulty of determining the point between the use of medicine as a tool of pacification and as a legitimate therapeutic aid for the treatment of the mentally incompetent. Obviously many cases will be clearly one or the other. However, there will be borderline cases where there is a risk of confusion between convenience to the prison administration and genuine medical need. We felt that this underlined the need for adequate review or appeal procedures.

We received evidence that doctors were frequently victimised for having undertaken professional and human rights activities ranging from protesting about inadequacies in the health system through to work carried out in human rights organizations. Any attempt to encourage doctors to oppose abuses will require us to address the risk they face. We believe that doctors in the front line need tangible and visible support — from their medical associations, from the world medical community and from other concerned organizations and individuals. We cannot demand of doctors a super-human dedication to preserving medical ethics in the face of gross repressive forces unless there is a concomitant level of support.

Unfortunately, medical associations in various countries have not responded to human rights violations involving doctors in a way which can inspire pride. In some cases this is because the medical association is a sham created by the government following the arrest of elected leaders. In other cases the association apparently does not feel any obligation to intervene on behalf of doctors arrested for "political" reasons or is disinterested for reasons that have more to do with apathy.

The Working Party commends the work done by human rights organizations on issues of deep importance to the medical community and expresses the hope that they will continue to give these issues their attention.

Recommendations

Involvement of doctors in torture

1   We entirely endorse the conclusion of the 1986 BMA *Torture Report*, that "torture or brutal treatment of detained persons corrupts society". We condemn such treatment regardless of

whether it occurs in prisons, police stations, other adult or juvenile residential centres or psychiatric institutions. *We strongly recommend that all establishments where individuals are detained by law or by circumstance should be open to inspection and comply with accepted humanitarian standards.* In this regard, we welcome the work of the European Committee for the Prevention of Torture and inhuman or degrading treatment or punishment and urge governments to work towards the establishment of an international equivalent.

2   Medicine confers both privileges and obligations. The practice of torture or other cruel, inhuman or degrading treatment is abhorrent and medical participation in such acts is particularly abhorrent. All citizens have a moral duty to oppose illegal brutality but in resisting the proliferation of ill-treatment, more is expected of the medical practitioner. *If the possibility of abuses of human rights comes to the attention of a medical practitioner they have an ethical duty to take immediate action. To fail to take an immediate stand on principle makes protest or withdrawal much more difficult at a later stage.*

3   All doctors carry responsibility for safeguarding the ethical practice of medicine. Prison doctors, Armed Forces doctors, and doctors employed in psychiatric facilities have a particular duty to be vigilant given the potential for abuse which occurs in these institutions. *Doctors have a particular duty to act when it is within their power, either individually or through their professional bodies, to exert a positive influence.*

4   We are deeply concerned by the evidence presented to us of doctors either participating in torture without qualm or turning a blind eye when it occurs. We have no hesitation in condemning the collaboration of doctors in maltreatment. While we have every sympathy with those who are put at risk by their refusal to co-operate in torture, collaboration with torturers in response to pressures such as fear of loss of jobs or status is unacceptable. *We recommend that the behaviour of practitioners who are alleged to take part in torture is fully and fairly investigated and that those found culpable are barred from medical practice and from membership of professional associations.*

5   It is wrong for a doctor to voluntarily participate in maltreatment even in the expectation of diminishing the damage to individuals.

Well-intentioned doctors who accept such a role may be unaware of the long-term psychological trauma and distress engendered by their presence. *If doctors are forced, by reason of severe threat to the safety of themselves or those close to them, to be present during ill-treatment or torture, or to treat a tortured prisoner without clinical freedom, they should report this fact to a responsible body.* It is for the doctor's judgment to decide what national body can be trusted to handle such information responsibly. In the absence of any national body which can receive such allegations, international support is needed. Appropriate bodies to receive such allegations would include the UN, the World Medical Association, the Commonwealth Medical Association (CMA), the International Committee of the Red Cross and Amnesty International.

6   *We urge responsible international bodies such as those mentioned above to investigate establishing a mechanism for reviewing and making known cases in which doctors have been involved in abuses of human rights and to determine the most appropriate international sanction which could be applied.*

Provision of medical care to prisoners and torture victims

7   When a doctor is called upon to treat a victim of torture after the event, the doctor must consider the prisoner's best interests as paramount. We are concerned that some people who have been tortured have been denied necessary medical care. *Medical treatment should be given to torture victims, subject to their consent, in an ethical manner; it is essential that (i) the doctor can act with clinical freedom; (ii) the doctor can identify himself or herself; (iii) the prisoner is identified or identifiable.*

8   *If the prisoner is unable to consent by reason of being unconscious or drugged, for example, medical care should be provided in accordance with the ethical guidelines which would cover any other acute case.*

9   In some cases where a prisoner had suffered ill-health following torture, the authorities' or doctor's refusal to give medical help was deliberate, malevolent and tantamount to a continuation of the torture. *We recommend that doctors refusing to give or to arrange adequate care to such prisoners should be subject to disciplinary action.*

Treatment of hunger-strikers

10 We received evidence of several cases where hunger-strikers had been forcibly fed with a view either to punishment or to avoiding possible embarrassment to the prison authorities which would be caused by prisoners' deaths. We reaffirm the Declaration of Tokyo, which states that where a prisoner refuses nourishment and is considered by the doctor as capable of forming an unimpaired and rational judgement concerning the consequences of such a voluntary refusal of nourishment, he or she shall not be fed artificially. *We recommend that artificial feeding and the way in which it is carried out must be a result of a clinical, and not an administrative, decision.*

11 *We recommend that doctors make their policy regarding resuscitation during hunger strike absolutely clear to the prisoner at the beginning of any strike. Doctors who feel unable for reasons of conscience, or for any other reason, to abide by the prisoner's decision must allow another doctor to supervise care.*

12 *A doctor who has any doubt about a prisoner's intention regarding hunger strikes, or who is asked to treat an unconscious prisoner whose wishes he cannot ascertain, must strive to do the best for that prisoner.* This might involve resuscitation if the prisoner's views are unknown. If, however, a doctor is clear and in no doubt about the prisoner's wish regarding resuscitation and feeding, he must respect it. If it is clear the prisoner intended to continue the strike until death, he must be allowed to die in dignity.

Doctors working in the Armed Forces, prisons and other non-civilian institutions

13 We received a great deal of evidence to suggest that, in many countries, doctors working in the prison service are viewed as an expert resource for controlling prisoners, rather than as medical professionals working for the benefit of their patients. *The contractual terms of prison doctors should acknowledge their professional independence to make clinical judgements. Doctors working in the prison system should be in a position to provide the same standards of medical care as is available to the general population.*

14 *Medical services in prisons should be separate from the prison officers' role of controlling or punishing prisoners. Prison medical officers must be able to offer independent clinical recommendations for treatment.*

15 *Doctors working in prisons must be able to keep independent confidential records.*

16 The Armed Services and the prison service are potentially coercive in nature, and are not medical institutions. For this reason, it is important that doctors working in these situations are able to appeal to an independent authority in the case of potential breaches of medical ethics. In the UK, doctors working in the Armed Forces have the right of appeal to the BMA's Ethics Committee if they are asked to do something which they feel is contrary to medical ethics. *We recommend that such an appeals procedure be extended to prisons and believe that the principle should apply in all military and prison services.*

Support for doctors entering the prison service and Armed Forces

17 The Working Party noted that, in many cases, it was a newcomer to a situation who raised questions about the treatment of detainees. At the same time, we were concerned that someone coming into an established situation was particularly vulnerable to pressure to conform to the prevailing culture. We heard that in the UK, during the first months after entering military service, doctors are given guidance on medical ethics. *We believe that this practice of providing ethical guidance in the Armed Forces should be adopted in other countries and recommend that it be extended to those working in the prison service in the UK.*

18 We were concerned that doctors working in closed communities such as prisons or mental hospitals may have few opportunities to broaden their experience and may thus be liable to suffer from professional stagnation. *We recommend that doctors working under these conditions in the UK should have the opportunity to rotate jobs so as to widen their perspective.*

Strengthening medical ethics

19 We felt that it was imperative that training in ethics should be strengthened in order to give doctors a framework in which to carry

out their medical practice. We believe that individual doctors would be more able to withstand pressures if they had been given clear ethical guidance at medical schools and in their post-graduate training. *We recommend that medical schools incorporate medical ethics into the core curriculum and that all medical graduates make a commitment, by means of affirmation, to observe an ethical code such as the WMA's International Code of Medical Ethics. We recommend that those national medical associations which have not already done so should adopt clear ethical guidelines and welcome the intention of the Commonwealth Medical Association to develop a code of ethics for doctors working in developing countries.*

20 We welcome the work of the General Medical Council in ensuring that standards of medical ethics are upheld in both education and practice and we support the efforts of that body to examine the standards of those from overseas seeking to practice here. However, we feel that there is room for improvement in the standards of medical ethics both here and worldwide. *We welcome any steps taken by the GMC to look carefully at the recognition of medical training, in whatever country it is undertaken, which does not include adequate instruction and examination in ethics.*

21 We reaffirm our commitment to the Declaration of Tokyo and to other international codes of practice and regret that the existing codes are not universally respected. We support the efforts of the Danish and Uruguayan Medical Associations and non-governmental bodies to develop clear and unambiguous codes. *We urge wider and more effective adherence to existing standards.*

Action by national medical associations

22 The Working Party was concerned to note that some national medical associations had not done enough to address allegations of medical involvement in torture in their countries. We feel strongly that national medical associations have a duty to investigate allegations and to speak out when doctors are found to take part in torture. *We recommend that all medical associations and disciplinary bodies adopt a declaration opposing the involvement of doctors in torture, and giving an undertaking to remove from their membership or registers any doctor found to be taking part in gross and illegal abuses of medical ethics.*

23   *We recommend to the BMA Council that any medical association apparently failing to take action on their members' involvement in torture should be asked to explain their apparent inaction.*

24   We reaffirm our support for the activities of the BMA in opposing medical involvement in torture as set out in annex 1. We welcome initiatives taken by other medical associations. *We appeal to the international medical community to encourage effective opposition to torture in countries where the pressure for medical participation in human rights violations is considerable.*

Doctors and the death penalty

25   We welcome the trend to limit the application of capital punishment. We believe that the active involvement of doctors in carrying out the death sentence is unethical. We do not believe that doctors have any place at an execution. *We recommend that all medical associations should adopt resolutions condemning active medical involvement in application of this punishment.*

26   In our opinion, certification of death is part of normal medical duties and that this extends to death by judicial execution. However, we were concerned about reports that medical professionals, while ostensibly attending executions as witnesses, had in fact monitored the execution process and given advice about whether or not the victim was dead and thus whether or not to repeat the execution process. *We strongly recommend that, where judicial executions are carried out, certification of death should take place away from the site of execution and several hours after it so that there is no doubt about life being extinct.*

27   While appreciating the sincere desire of doctors to alleviate the shortage of human organs for transplantation, we deplore the practice of using organs from executed prisoners for this purpose. We have no objection to transplants provided that free consent can be given, but condemned prisoners are not in a position to give free consent. There is a danger that decisions about whether or not to impose the death penalty or to allow appeals may be influenced by the possibility of obtaining organs for donation. We support the work the GMC is doing in this area and urge it to include guidance on the use of organs in such circumstances in future published standards. *We would like to see the GMC adopt a policy to address cases of any surgeons found to be involved in the removal of organs*

from executed prisoners for use in transplants, and recommend that it discuss appropriate measures to be taken against those knowingly using organs taken from executed prisoners by others. We call on national medical associations, the UK Royal Colleges and other similar organizations to communicate their opposition in the strongest terms to any medical body which condones this practice.

28   We do not consider that giving forensic medical evidence to help determine guilt or innocence at a capital trial is different in substance to giving evidence for such purposes at other trials and therefore believe that giving evidence of fact is non-problematic (though some might find it distasteful). However, we believe that doctors should not certify prisoners fit for any procedure which would be detrimental to their interests. *Providing medical opinion on "fitness for execution" is not an appropriate role for medical practitioners.*

29   A just society rightly prohibits the execution of people who are mentally ill. We are concerned that in some countries ethically acceptable measures have not been developed to take account of those whose mental health significantly deteriorates while they are awaiting execution. The Working Party has strong reservations about the practice of treating mentally ill patients so as to render them "fit for execution". Attempting to provide rehabilitation and treatment for a prisoner who will be executed upon improvement of his mental illness puts medical professionals in an intolerable situation. *We recommend that prisoners who have become mentally ill while under sentence of death should have their sentences commuted to allow for normal rehabilitative treatment to take place in an ethical manner.*

30   We find the idea of giving emergency life-saving medical care to prisoners awaiting execution, solely to keep them alive until execution is carried out, bizarre and abhorrent. *We recommend that doctors place emphasis on the fact that prisoners under sentence of death have complete rights to adequate medical care which should be given with due respect to the prisoner's right to grant or withhold consent.*

Whipping and amputations

31   The Working Party felt that doctors who were asked to superintend the administration of, to carry out or to certify prisoners fit for

corporal punishment were put into an invidious position. In carrying out the sentence of amputation, the physical suffering of an individual could be lessened if a doctor performs the procedure. Conversely, participation of a doctor in judicial corporal punishment does not necessarily prevent severe psychological or physical suffering and death or permanent mutilation of the victim. Medical participation gives a spurious humanity to corporal punishment. *Having given careful consideration to both sides of the argument, we firmly recommend that doctors should not participate in corporal punishment either by certifying fitness or by performing amputations.*

32   Doctors should not become part of the penal system. If governments choose to carry out life-threatening punishments, they must not look to the medical profession to alleviate or contain the suffering so imposed. In the long-term we believe that medical participation is detrimental. We received evidence that refusal to participate may reduce the number of sentences carried out. In Pakistan, doctors have effectively prevented the carrying out of judicial amputations by their refusal to take part. *We recommend that professional associations and individual doctors make clear their opposition to such punishments.*

33   In some countries, for example the Netherlands, health workers who undertake service abroad receive specific guidance on participation in judicial punishments. They are also given a written policy statement to hand to any authority requiring them to take part in corporal punishments. This guidance draws attention to international standards and the policy that Dutch doctors will not certify prisoners fit for punishment or participate in any way in judicial punishments or executions. On each occasion that the health worker is asked to participate in such procedures by local authorities, he or she explains the objections to so doing. In this way, the doctor is protected from taking part in the punishment, and also draws the attention of colleagues in the country to international opinion on the matter. *We recommend that this procedure be adopted more widely as a measure to protect the doctor and to help combat medical involvement in these punishments and eventually to discourage the punishments themselves. We believe that the UK government should make clear its opposition to the involvement of British doctors working abroad in such punishments.*

The role of forensic medicine

34   We were impressed by the number of cases in which accurate and dispassionate forensic medical evidence contributed to strengthening the hands of those seeking justice in the wake of human rights violations. The new United Nations standard on the investigation of deaths is welcome and deserves widespread dissemination. Examples of false, inadequate or absent forensic statements are often the result of inadequate forensic training. We commend the teaching program of the American Association for the Advancement of Science which currently offers training to doctors who might be able to apply new skills to the protection of human rights in their own countries. *We recommend that the World Health Organization, the UN Division of Criminal Justice and the UN Human Rights Commission should investigate the possibility of organizing a similar training project.*

35   We were equally and negatively struck by the number of examples of false, inadequate and absent forensic statements brought to our attention. *We recommend that medical associations should investigate alleged failures of forensic specialists and discipline those who deliberately produce false certificates. Equally importantly, there is a need to support forensic staff who are under pressure to falsify their findings.*

Protection of health professionals

36   The Working Party strongly endorsed the actions of the BMA in upholding the ethical practice of medicine, protecting human rights and supporting doctors who protest about abuses of medical training. *We recommend that the Association should continue this work and that it should maintain a dialogue on human rights and medical issues with sister associations to maximise the effectiveness of actions which each undertakes.*

37   We believe that the risks faced by doctors in areas with poor human rights records needs to be more widely recognized. It was clear to us that demanding that doctors respect medical ethics is meaningless if they are not given leadership and support in facing the risks they incur as a result of taking a firm stand. *We recommend that national and international medical bodies such as the major international professional associations should develop and give publicity to practical measures which can be taken to support*

individual doctors and medical associations which face repression for their professional or human rights activities.

38 We believe that the United Nations and its agencies such as the Human Rights Commission have an important role to play in monitoring abuses against medical personnel and feeding that information into the protective work they undertake. *We recommend that the UN human rights agencies monitor such abuses and develop a mechanism to protect medical personnel at risk as a result of their professional activities.*

Care for victims of human rights violations

39 We strongly support the development of social and health services for individuals who have been tortured and for the families who must cope with the effects of torture and exile. While expressing the strongest admiration and encouragement to those centres currently carrying out their difficult but invaluable work, we recognize that the scale of the human rights problem is such that small and over-stretched centres are unlikely to be able to cope by themselves. *We urge that the national medical associations in countries where such centres exist support this work, through publicity, material aid and any other means they find appropriate.* In addition, we feel that governments have a responsibility to devote sufficient resources to permit the mainstream health system to cope with the needs of this group of people.

40 The London-based Medical Foundation for the Care of Victims of Torture welcomes professional volunteers to treat torture victims and their families and to prepare medical reports documenting evidence of torture at the request of asylum-seekers' legal representatives. *We urge our members to consider this valuable area of voluntary work. In addition, we bring to the attention of our members in general practice the needs of asylum seekers and refugees, many of whom have been tortured and some of whom have language difficulties.*

41 In Britain, agencies such as the Medical Foundation for the Care of Victims of Torture have repeatedly drawn attention to inadequacies in the reception and appraisal procedures for asylum seekers and their families who claim to have suffered maltreatment or torture. We consider it extremely regrettable that in many countries, including the UK, asylum seekers are virtually criminalised. *We*

urge the government to ensure that accommodation and medical treatment outside the prison system can be provided for all those seeking asylum.

42 *We recommend that doctors treating detained asylum seekers make a full and careful record of any sign of injury on the first occasion of meeting the prisoner, or at the earliest opportunity.* Such a record may later be helpful in assessing applications for refugee status.

43 *When it is considered necessary, exceptionally, to detain asylum seekers, access to interpreters must be provided so that they can fully understand what is happening to them. Medical assessment and treatment should ideally be provided by doctors experienced in their problems.*

44 We are concerned that some asylum seekers who have suffered torture are being returned to their countries of origin because adequate evidence of their abuse has not been available. *We recommend that resources be provided so that information about the physical and psychological signs and symptoms of torture gathered by organizations in this field, for example the Medical Foundation for the Care of Victims of Torture, be made available to medical practitioners in the UK, with priority being given to those working in areas receiving refugees*[3].

Other issues

45 In this report, we have identified human rights issues involving medical participation which we do not feel fall within our own remit. The Working Party is anxious, however, that such issues should not be ignored. *We recommend that the BMA establish a Working Party to examine the issues we have drawn attention to but to which we were unable to give full attention, particularly the unacceptable standards prevailing in some British residential facilities and psychogeriatric institutions.*

---

3 Available literature, as well as information about existing centres, is cited in Gruschow J, Hannibal K. *Health Services for the Treatment of Torture and Trauma Survivors*. Washington DC: AAAS, 1990; *Selected bibliography on the health professions and human rights*. AI Index: ACT 75/06/90, 1990.

Further action

46 In the six years since the publication of the BMA's first Torture
Report, there have been major political upheavals and the map of
the world is changing rapidly. Despite much encouraging progress
in the field of human rights, we found incontrovertible evidence
that doctors are still involved both actively and passively in brutal
abuses. We strongly believe that the BMA, as one of the major
medical associations, has an important part to play in the protection
of human rights. *We recommend that the BMA medical ethics
committee keep this matter constantly under review and we urge the
Association to set up a panel in five years' time to monitor the
implementation of the recommendations set out in this report.*

Appendices

Appendix 1. *BMA procedures for human rights interventions*

1. The BMA does not have the capacity to verify all information submitted to it. Any information received must be verified with Amnesty International (AI) before a case is pursued. *No case* in which AI believes there to be a significant element of doubt should be pursued.

2. Information reported by groups other than AI and not already available to AI, will be forwarded to that organization for its investigation. *No action* can be taken until the information has been verified.

3. If reputable bodies in the same country as the potential human rights case are in a position to verify evidence or support the BMA's own request for further information, it may be decided to request their assistance. This can only be done after discussion with the Head of Division and obtaining advice from regional experts regarding the potential danger to any of the parties involved.

4. The BMA will only consider cases in which doctors are involved. For example:

- Doctors may be involved because of their participation in activities contrary to the Declaration of Tokyo such as the forced feeding of hunger-strikers.
- Doctors may be involved in practices contrary to the recommendations of the BMA Torture Report such as monitoring torture, examining fitness for torture, or administration of capital punishment.
- Doctors may themselves be victims of human rights abuses.

5. Cases of alleged human rights abuses in which doctors are not directly involved *will not* be pursued. These include repressive measures against patients, kidnapping of patients, military interference with provision of medical services, discrimination in provision of medical care abroad and restriction in the provision of medical care to prisoners abroad.

6. Even where information has been substantiated by reputable agencies such as AI, the BMA will not make any accusations but will request information or assistance in establishing the circumstances.

7. Letters of enquiry should normally be directed to the relevant medical association requesting assistance in eliciting information.

8. Where there is no national medical association, letters of enquiry will be sent either to the Minister of Health or the Head of State, urging that the matter be clarified. The Association may draw attention to the allegations which have been raised and request that they be looked into.

9. Where the national medical association is itself the object of repression, advice will be taken from regional experts as to whether contact with that association would pose a danger to it. If it is not considered to pose a danger, or at the specific request of the national medical association, the BMA may address letters of enquiry to the Minister of Health or Head of State, urging that the matter be clarified and international legal instruments observed.

10 *Under no circumstances* will the BMA request the immediate or unconditional release of any detained person. For those in long-term detention without trial, the BMA may request that any intended charges be brought and the detainee granted a fair trial under the provision of international legal instruments.

Appendix 2. *Resolutions passed by BMA Annual Representative Meetings (ARM)*

Chile
That this Meeting supports exiled Chilean doctors who wish to return to live and work in their native land. (1986)

Confidentiality
That there should be no intrusion into the secrecy of the transaction between patient and doctor except:
1. with the full and informed consent of the patient, or
2. by order of a judge in open court as at present. (1983)

Degrading treatment
That this Meeting unequivocally condemns the usage of medical personnel in enforcement of inhuman laws and degrading measures. (1981)

Female circumcision
That BMA supports legislation outlawing "female circumcision" except where a disease process is present. (1983)

Intimate body searches
That this Meeting believes that no medical practitioner should take part in an intimate body search of a subject without that subject's consent. (1989)

Political beliefs

That this Meeting deplores any regime taking actions against doctors simply because of the political beliefs of their patients whom they are bound to treat in the cause of common humanity and according to the International Code of Medical Ethics. (1978)

Political prisoners

That this Representative Body deplores the continued abuse of medical skills and ethics for political ends in contravention of the principles of the Declaration of Geneva. (1976)

South Africa

That this Meeting urges the Medical Association of South Africa to do everything possible to install the colour equality of all members of the medical profession in South Africa. (1972)

That this Meeting recognizes that there is racial discrimination in health care in South Africa and:

(a) calls on BMA members to refrain from visiting any medical institution which is practising apartheid in that country;

(b) views with concern the problems facing doctors in that country. (1986)

That this Meeting urges Council to take a public stand against any form of apartheid practice on health care, support the policies of National Medical and Dental Association (NAMDA), and demand the release of Dr Ivan Toms, imprisoned in the Republic of South Africa for refusing to take up arms to sustain apartheid. (1988)

Soviet Union — Free movement

That this Meeting is gravely concerned by the plight of some 200 Jewish doctors in the Soviet Union who have been refused the right to emigrate and demands that the Soviet Union should abide by the Helsinki Agreement in respect of the free movement of its citizens. (1984)

That this Meeting denounces the practice current in the Soviet Union of denying necessary medical care to prisoners of conscience and to those refused the right to emigrate and demands that this practice should cease. (1984)

That this Meeting is gravely concerned at the apparent deterioration in the health care of political prisoners and asks Council to campaign on this issue. (1987)

Teaching of medical ethics

That this Meeting requests the GMC to instruct medical schools to have an identifiable, substantial part of the undergraduate medical curriculum devoted to the ethical and legal aspects of medical practice and that such teaching should be introduced in a non-dogmatic manner. (1986)

Torture
That this Meeting endorses, in full, the Declaration of Tokyo 1975 of the WMA. (1979)

That this Meeting reaffirms that medical ethics prohibit medical involvement in torture and supports resistance offered by doctors and their medical associations to the use of torture. (1984)

That this Meeting requests Council to set up a working party to investigate claims that, in some countries, doctors are co-operating with the use of torture as a routine instrument of repression by governments of all political persuasions. (1984)

That this Meeting strongly supports the view of the Working Party on Torture that it is important to maintain a proper distance between the medical profession and the apparatus of the state and recommends that:

(a)   the BMA should provide support whenever possible both to medical associations and to individual doctors in this country and abroad, who are faced with problems of conscience or believe they have evidence of torture and need help.

(b)   the BMA should make provision for professional censure of medical associations which acquiesce in torture. (1986)

That this Meeting views with great concern continuing reports of the abuses of medical skills in relation to prisoners, and asks Council to establish a working party to follow-up the torture report, to examine new evidence, and to make appropriate recommendations. (1989)

Appendix 3. *Declaration of Tokyo* (World Medical Association, 1975)

It is the privilege of the medical doctor to practise medicine in the service of humanity, to preserve and restore bodily and mental health without distinction as to the person's comfort and to ease the suffering of his or her patients. The utmost respect for human life is to be maintained even under threat, and no use made of any medical knowledge contrary to the laws of humanity.

For the purpose of this Declaration, torture is defined as the deliberate, systematic, wanton infliction of physical or mental suffering by one or more persons acting alone or on the authority or any authority, to force another person to yield information, to make a confession, or for any other reason.

1. The doctor shall not countenance, condone or participate in the practice of torture or other forms of cruel, inhuman or degrading procedures, whatever the offence of which the victim of such procedures is

suspected, accused or guilty, and whatever the victim's beliefs or motives, and in all situations, including armed conflict and civil strife.

2. The doctor shall not provide any premises, instruments, substances or knowledge to facilitate the practice of torture or other forms of cruel, inhuman or degrading treatment or to diminish the ability of the victim to resist such treatment.

3. The doctor shall not be present during any procedure during which torture or other forms of cruel, inhuman or degrading treatment is used or threatened.

4. A doctor must have complete clinical independence in deciding upon the care of a person for whom he or she is medically responsible. The doctor's fundamental role is to alleviate the distress of his or her fellow men, and no motive, whether personal, collective or political, shall prevail against this higher purpose.

5. Where a prisoner refuses nourishment and is considered by the doctor as capable of forming unimpaired and rational judgement concerning the consequences of such a voluntary refusal of nourishment, he or she shall not be fed artificially. The decision as to the capacity of the prisoner to form such a judgement should be confirmed by at least one other independent doctor. The consequences of the refusal of such nourishment shall be explained by the doctor to the prisoner.

6. The World Medical Association will support, and should encourage, the international community, the national medical associations and fellow doctors, to support the doctor and his or her family in the face of threats or reprisals resulting from a refusal to condone the use of torture or other form of cruel, inhuman or degrading treatment.

Appendix 4. *WMA resolution on physician participation in capital punishment (1981)*

Resolved, that the assembly of the World Medical Association endorses the action of the Secretary-General in issuing the attached press release on behalf of the World Medical Association condemning physician participation in capital punishment.

Further resolved, that it is unethical for physicians to participate in capital punishment, although this does not preclude physicians certifying death.

Further resolved, that the [WMA] Medical Ethics Committee keep the matter under active consideration.

Secretary-General's Press Release

The first capital punishment by intravenous injection of lethal dose of drugs was decided to be carried out next week by the court of the State of Oklahoma, USA.

Regardless of the method of capital punishment a state imposes, no physician should be required to be an active participant. Physicians are dedicated to preserving life.

Acting as an executioner is not the practice of medicine, and physician services are not required to carry out capital punishment even if the methodology utilizes pharmacological agents or equipment that might otherwise be used in the practice of medicine.

A physician's role would be to certify death once the state had carried out the capital punishment.

September 11, 1981

Appendix 5. *WMA Declaration on Hunger-Strikers (1991)*

Preamble

1. The doctor treating hunger-strikers is faced with the following conflicting values:

    1.1 There is a moral obligation on every human being to respect the sanctity of life. This is especially evident in the case of a doctor who exercises his skills to save life and also acts in the best interests of his patients (beneficence).

    1.2 It is the duty of the doctor to respect the autonomy which the patient has over his person. A doctor requires informed consent from his patients before applying any of his skills to assist them, unless emergency circumstances have arisen in which case the doctor has to act in what is perceived to be the patient's best interests.

2. This conflict is apparent where a hunger-striker who has issued clear instruction not to be resuscitated lapses into a coma and is about to die. Moral obligation urges the doctor to resuscitate the patient even though it is against the patient's wishes. On the other hand, duty urges the doctor to respect the autonomy of the patient.

    2.1 Ruling in favour of intervention may undermine the autonomy which the patient has over himself.

2.2 Ruling in favour of non-intervention may result in a doctor having to face the tragedy of an avoidable death.

3. A doctor/patient relationship is said to be in existence whenever a doctor is duty bound, by virtue of his obligation to the patient, to apply his skills to any person, be it in the form of advice or treatment.

   This relationship can exist in spite of the fact that the patient might not consent [to] certain forms of treatment or intervention.

   Once the doctor agrees to attend to a hunger-striker, that person becomes the doctor's patient. This has all the implications and responsibilities inherent in the doctor/patient relationship, including consent and responsibility.

4. The ultimate decision on intervention or non-intervention should be left with the individual doctor without the intervention of third parties whose primary interest is not the patient's welfare. However, the doctor should clearly state to the patient whether or not he is able to accept the patient's decision to refuse treatment or, in case of coma, artificial feeding, thereby risking death. If the doctor cannot accept the patient's decision to refuse such aid, the patient would then be entitled to be attended by another physician.

Guidelines for the management of hunger-strikers

Since the medical profession considers the principle of sanctity of life to be fundamental to its practice, the following practical guidelines are recommended for doctors who treat hunger-strikers:

1. *Definition*
   A hunger-striker is a mentally competent person who has indicated that he has decided to embark on a hunger strike and has refused to take food and/or fluids for a significant interval.

2. *Ethical behaviour*
   2.1 A doctor should acquire a detailed medical history of the patient where possible.
   2.2 A doctor should carry out a thorough examination of the patient at the onset of the hunger strike.
   2.3 Doctors or other health care personnel may not apply undue pressure of any sort on the hunger-striker to suspend the strike. Treatment or care of the hunger-striker must not be conditional upon him suspending his hunger strike.
   2.4 The hunger-striker must be professionally informed by the doctor of the clinical consequences of a hunger strike, and of any specific

danger to his own particular case. An informed decision can only be made on the basis of clear communication. An interpreter should be used if indicated.

2.5 Should a hunger-striker wish to have a second medical opinion, this should be granted. Should a hunger-striker prefer his treatment to be continued by the second doctor, this should be permitted. In the case of the hunger-striker being a prisoner, this should be permitted by arrangement and consultation with the appointed prison doctor.

2.6 Treating infections or advising the patient to increase his oral intake of fluid (or accept intravenous saline solutions) is often acceptable to a hunger-striker. A refusal to accept such intervention must not prejudice any other aspect of the patient's health care. Any treatment administered to the patient must be with his approval.

3. *Clear instructions*
The doctor should ascertain on a daily basis whether or not the patient wishes to continue with his hunger strike. The doctor should also ascertain on a daily basis what the patient's wishes are with regard to treatment should he become unable to make an informed decision. These findings must be recorded in the doctor's personal medical records and kept confidential.

4. *Artificial feeding*
When the hunger-striker has become confused and is therefore unable to make an unimpaired decision or has lapsed into a coma, the doctor shall be free to make the decision for his patient as to further treatment which he considers to be in the best interest of that patient, always taking into account the decision he has arrived at during his preceding care of the patient during his hunger strike, and reaffirming article 4 of the preamble of this declaration.

5. *Coercion*
Hunger-strikers should be protected from coercive participation. This may require removal from the presence of fellow strikers.

6. *Family*
The doctor has a responsibility to inform the family of the patient that the patient has embarked on a hunger strike, unless this is specifically prohibited by the patient.

Appendix 6. *Declaration of Hawaii (WPA, 1977, 1983)*

Ever since the dawn of culture, ethics has been an essential part of the healing art. It is the view of the World Psychiatric Association that due to conflicting loyalties and expectations of both physicians and patients in contemporary society and the delicate nature of the therapist-patient relationship, high ethical standards are especially important for those involved in the science and practice of psychiatry as a medical specialty. These guidelines have been delineated in order to promote close adherence to those standards and to prevent misuse of psychiatric concepts, knowledge and technology.

Since the psychiatrist is a member of society as well as a practitioner of medicine, he or she must consider the ethical implications specific to psychiatry as well as the ethical demands of all physicians and the social responsibility of every man and woman.

Even though ethical behaviour is based on the individual psychiatrist's conscience and personal judgement, written guidelines are needed to clarify the profession's ethical implications.

Therefore, the General Assembly of the World Psychiatric Association has approved these ethical guidelines for psychiatrists, having in mind the great differences in cultural backgrounds, and in legal, social and economic conditions which exist in the various countries in the world. It should be understood that the World Psychiatric Association views these guidelines to be minimal requirements for the ethical standards of the psychiatric profession.

1. The aim of psychiatry is to treat mental illness and to promote mental health. To the best of his or her ability, consistent with accepted scientific knowledge and ethical principles, the psychiatrist shall serve the best interests of the patient and be also concerned for the common good and a just allocation of health resources. To fulfil these aims requires continuous research and continual education of health care personnel, patients and public.

2. Every psychiatrist should offer to the patient the best available therapy to his knowledge and if accepted must treat him or her with the solicitude and respect due to the dignity of all human beings. When the psychiatrist is responsible for treatment given by others he owes them competent supervision and education. Whenever there is a need, or whenever a reasonable request is forthcoming from the patient, the psychiatrist should seek the help of anther colleague.

3. The psychiatrist aspires for a therapeutic relationship that is founded on mutual agreement. At its optimum it requires trust, confidentiality, co-operation and mutual responsibility. Such a relationship may not be possible to establish with some patients. In that case, contact should be established

with a relative or other person close to the patient. If and when a relationship is established for purposes other than therapeutic, such as in forensic psychiatry, its nature must be thoroughly explained to the person concerned.

4. The psychiatrist should inform the patient of the nature of the condition, therapeutic procedures, including possible alternatives, and of the possible outcome. This information must be afforded in a considerate way and the patient must be given the opportunity to choose between appropriate and available methods.

5. No procedure shall be performed nor treatment given against or independent of a patient's own will, unless, because of mental illness, the patient cannot form a judgement as to what is in his or her best interests and without which treatment serious impairment is likely to occur to the patient or others.

6. As soon as the conditions for compulsory treatment no longer apply, the psychiatrist should release the patient from the compulsory nature of the treatment and if further therapy is necessary should obtain voluntary consent. The psychiatrist should inform the patient, and/or relatives or meaningful others, of the existence of mechanisms of appeal for the detention and for any other complaints related to his or her well-being.

7. The psychiatrist must never use his professional possibilities to violate the dignity of human rights of any individual or group and should never let inappropriate personal desires, feelings, prejudices or beliefs interfere with the treatment. The psychiatrist must on no account utilize the tool of his profession, once the absence of psychiatric illness has been established. If a patient or some third party demands actions contrary to scientific knowledge or ethical principles the psychiatrist must refuse to cooperate.

8. Whatever the psychiatrist has been told by the patient, or has noted during examination or treatment, must be kept confidential unless the patient relieves the psychiatrist from this obligation, or to prevent serious harm to self or others makes disclosure necessary. In these cases, however, the patient should be informed of the breach of confidentiality.

9. To increase and propagate psychiatric knowledge and skill requires participation of the patients. Informed consent must, however, be obtained before presenting a patient to a class and, if possible, also when a case history is released for scientific publication, whereby all reasonable measures must be taken to preserve the dignity and anonymity of the patient and to safeguard the personal reputation of the subject. The patient's participation must be voluntary, after full information has been given for the aim, procedures, risks and inconveniences of a research project and there must always be a reasonable relationship between calculated risks or inconvenience and the benefit of the study. In clinical research every subject must retain and exert his rights as a patient. For children and other patients who cannot themselves give informed consent, this should be obtained from

the legal next-of-kin. Every patient or research subject is free to withdraw for any reason at any time from any voluntary treatment and from any teaching or research program in which he or she participates. This withdrawal, as well as any refusal to enter a program, must never influence the psychiatrist's efforts to help the patient or subject.

10. The psychiatrist should stop all therapeutic, teaching or research programs that may evolve contrary to the principles of this Declaration.

Appendix 7. *Declaration on the Participation of Psychiatrists in the Death Penalty (WPA, 1989)*

Psychiatrists are physicians and adhere to the Hippocratic Oath "to practise for the good of their patients and never to do harm".

The World Psychiatric Association is an international association with 77 Member Societies.

Considering that the United Nations' Principles of Medical Ethics enjoins physicians — and thus psychiatrists — to refuse to enter into any relationship with a prisoner other than one directed at evaluating, protecting or improving their physical and mental health, and further

Considering that the Declaration of Hawaii of the WPA resolves that the psychiatrist shall serve the best interests of the patient and treat every patient with the solicitude and respect due to the dignity of all human beings and that the psychiatrist must refuse to cooperate if some third party demands actions contrary to ethical principles,

Conscious that psychiatrists may be called on to participate in any action connected to executions,

Declares that the participation of psychiatrists in any such action is a violation of professional ethics.

Appendix 8. *United Nations Principles of Medical Ethics (1982)*

The General Assembly...*

Desirous of setting further standards in this field which ought to be implemented by health personnel, particularly physicians, and by government officials,

---

* The preamble to this resolution has been edited. For the full text see UN document A/RES/37/194.

1. Adopts the Principles of Medical Ethics relevant to the role of health personnel, particularly physicians, in the protection of prisoners and detainees against torture and other cruel, inhuman or degrading treatment or punishment set forth in the annex to the present resolution;

2. Calls upon all Governments to give the Principles of Medical Ethics, together with the present resolution, the widest possible distribution, in particular among medical and paramedical associations and institutions of detention or imprisonment in an official language of the state;

3. Invites all relevant inter-governmental organizations, in particular the World Health Organization, and non-governmental organizations concerned to bring the Principles of Medical Ethics to the attention of the widest possible group of individuals, especially those active in the medical or paramedical field.

Principles of Medical Ethics Relevant to the Role of Health Personnel, particularly Physicians, in the Protection of Prisoners and Detainees against Torture and other Cruel, Inhuman or Degrading Treatment or Punishment.

Principle 1

Health personnel, especially physicians, charged with the medical care of prisoners and detainees have the duty to provide them with protection of their physical and mental health and treatment of disease of the same quality and standard as is afforded to those who are not imprisoned or detained.

Principle 2

It is a gross contravention of medical ethics, as well as an offence under applicable international instruments, for health personnel, particularly physicians, to engage, actively or passively, in acts which constitute participation in, complicity in, incitement to or attempts to commit torture or other cruel, inhuman or degrading treatment or punishment.[1]

---

1   See the Declaration on the Protection of All Persons from Being Subjected to Torture and Other Cruel, Inhuman or Degrading Treatment or Punishment (General Assembly Resolution 3452 (xxx), annex), article 1 of which states:

"1. For the purpose of this Declaration, torture means any act by which severe pain or suffering, whether physical or mental, is intentionally inflicted by or at the instigation of a public official on a person for such purposes as obtaining from him or a third person information or confession, punishing him for an act he has committed or is suspected of having committed, or intimidating him or other persons. It does not include pain or suffering arising only from, inherent or incidental to, lawful sanctions to the extent consistent with the Standard

Principle 3

It is a contravention of medical ethics for health personnel, particularly physicians, to be involved in any professional relationship with prisoners or detainees the purpose of which is not to solely evaluate, protect or improve their physical and mental health.

Principle 4

It is a contravention of medical ethics for health personnel, particularly physicians:

a) to apply their knowledge and skills in order to assist in the interrogation of prisoners and detainees in a manner that may adversely affect the physical or mental health of such prisoners or detainees and which is not in accordance with the relevant international instruments.[2]

b) To certify, or to participate in the certification of, the fitness of prisoners or detainees for any form of treatment or punishment that may adversely affect their physical or mental health and which is not in accordance with the relevant international instruments, or to participate in any way in the infliction of such treatment or punishment which is not in accordance with the relevant international instruments.

Principle 5

It is a contravention of medical ethics for health personnel, particularly physicians, to participate in any procedure for restraining a prisoner or detainee unless such a procedure is determined in accordance with purely medical criteria as being necessary for the protection of the physical or

---

Minimum Rules for the Treatment of Prisoners.

2. Torture constitutes an aggravated and deliberate form of cruel, inhuman or degrading treatment or punishment."

Article 7 of the Declaration states:

"Each state shall ensure that all acts of torture as defined in article 1 are offenses under its criminal law. The same shall apply in regard to acts which constitute participation in, complicity in, incitement to or an attempt to commit torture."

2 Particularly the Universal Declaration of Human Rights (General Assembly resolution 217 A (III)), the International Covenants on Human Rights (General Assembly Resolution 3452 (xxx), annex) and the Standard Minimum Rules for the Treatment of Prisoners (First United Nations Congress on the Prevention of Crime and the Treatment of Offenders: report by the Secretariat (United Nations publication, sales No. 1956.IV.4), annex IA).

mental health or the safety of the prisoner or detainee himself, or his fellow prisoners or detainees, or of his guardians, and presents no hazard to his physical or mental health.

Principle 6

There may be no derogation from the foregoing principles on any grounds whatsoever, including public emergency.

Appendix 9. *Amnesty International's 12-point program for the prevention of torture (1983)*

Amnesty International calls on all governments to implement the following 12-Point Program for the Prevention of Torture. It invites concerned individuals and organizations to join in promoting the program. Amnesty International believes that the implementation of these measures is a positive indication of a government's commitment to abolish torture and to work for its abolition worldwide.

1. **Official condemnation of torture**. The highest authorities of every country should demonstrate their total opposition to torture. They should make clear to all law enforcement personnel that torture will not be tolerated under any circumstances.

2. **Limits on incommunicado detention**. Torture often takes place while the victims are held incommunicado - unable to contact people outside who could help them or find out what is happening to them. Governments should adopt safeguards to ensure that incommunicado detention does not become an opportunity for torture. It is vital that all prisoners be brought before a judicial authority promptly after being taken into custody and that relatives, lawyers and doctors have prompt and regular access to them.

3. **No secret detention**. In some countries torture takes place in secret centres, often after the victims are made to "disappear". Governments should ensure that prisoners are held in publicly recognized places, and that accurate information about their whereabouts is made available to relatives and lawyers.

4. **Safeguards during interrogation and custody**. Governments should keep procedures for detention and interrogation under regular review. All prisoners should be promptly told of their rights, including the right to lodge complaints about their treatment. There should be regular independent visits of inspection to places of detention. An important safeguard against torture would be the separation of authorities responsible for detention from those in charge of interrogation.

5. **Independent investigation of reports of torture**. Governments should ensure that all complaints and reports of torture are impartially and effectively investigated. The methods and findings of such investigations should be made public. Complainants and witnesses should be protected from intimidation.

6. **No use of statements extracted under torture**. Governments should ensure that confessions or other evidence obtained through torture may never be invoked in legal proceedings.

7. **Prohibition of torture in law**. Governments should ensure that acts of torture are punishable offenses under the criminal law. In accordance with international law, the prohibition of torture must not be suspended under any circumstances, including states of war or other public emergency.

8. **Prosecution of alleged torturers**. Those responsible for torture should be brought to justice. This principle should apply wherever they happen to be, wherever the crime was committed and whatever the nationality of the perpetrators or victims. There should be no "safe haven" for torturers.

9. **Training procedures**. It should be made clear during the training of all officials involved in the custody, interrogation or treatment of prisoners that torture is a criminal act. They should be instructed that they are obliged to refuse to obey any order to torture.

10. **Compensation and rehabilitation**. Victims of torture and their dependants should be entitled to obtain financial compensation. Victims should be provided with appropriate medical care or rehabilitation.

11. **International response**. Governments should use all available channels to intercede with governments accused of torture. Intergovernmental mechanisms should be established and used to investigate reports of torture urgently and to take effective action against it. Governments should ensure that military, security or police transfers or training do not facilitate the practice of torture.

12. **Ratification of international instruments**. All governments should ratify international instruments containing safeguards and remedies against torture, including the International Covenant on Civil and Political Rights and its Optional Protocol which provides for individual complaints.

Appendix 10. *Ratification of international conventions by UK governments*

International treaties, covenants, conventions and protocols come into force in the following way. They are first introduced for signature, a step by which a government signals its support for the existence of the standard without necessarily committing itself to be bound by its provisions. Once a treaty has gained a minimum number of signatures it enters into force and can then be ratified. Alternately, a state can combine signature and ratification by *acceding* to a treaty. Some conventions allow for states to declare derogations from the whole document as well as temporary derogations from certain provisions (as the UK has done on a rather extended temporary basis under the Prevention of Terrorism Act). In some cases, optional protocols adding to the initial document are opened for signature and ratification.

International and regional human rights treaties

International Covenant on Civil and Political Rights (ICCPR), 1966.
Came into force: 23 March 1976; *Ratified by UK:* 20 May 1976.

Optional protocol to ICCPR (allowing individual complaints to Human Rights Committee).
Came into force: 23 March 1976; *Not signed by UK.*

Second optional protocol to ICCPR (aiming at abolition of the death penalty)
Came into force: 11 July 1991; *Not signed by UK.*

Convention against torture and other cruel, inhuman or degrading treatment or punishment, 1984.
Came into force: 26 June 1987; *Ratified by UK:* 8 December 1988.

Convention on the Rights of the Child, 1989.
Came into force: 2 September 1990; *Ratified by UK:* 16 December 1991.

European Convention on Human Rights, 1950.
Came into force: 3 September 1953; *Ratified by UK* [3]*:* 8 March 1951.

European Convention for the Prevention of Torture and Inhuman or Degrading Treatment or Punishment, 1987.
Came into force: 1 February 1989; *Ratified by UK:* 24 June 1988.

Geneva Conventions of 12 August 1949.
Came into force: 21 October 1950; *Ratified by UK:* 23 September 1957.

Protocols I and II of Geneva Conventions, 1977.
Came into force: 7 December 1978; *Signed by UK but not ratified.*

---

3   On 14 November 1989, the UK announced its derogation from Article 5(3) of the European Convention on Human Rights which requires that a detainee be promptly charged or released. This followed a ruling by the European Court of Human Rights which found the UK government to be in breach of the Convention as a result of the application of the Prevention of Terrorism Act.

Bibliography

The following books and major reports are some of the sources for background information for this report. In addition many individual papers, articles and books have been cited in footnotes.

Amnesty International. *Argentina: Doctor convicted of torture released under "due obedience" law*. AI Index: AMR 13/10/87, 17 December 1987.

Amnesty International. *Chile: Evidence of torture*. London: Amnesty International, 1983.

Amnesty International. *Human rights in Chile: the role of the medical profession*. London: AI Index: AMR 22/36/86.

Amnesty International. *Torture in Greece: The first torturer's trial 1975*. London: Amnesty International, 1977.

Amnesty International. *Summary of Selected International Procedures and Bodies Dealing with Human Rights Matters*. AI Index: IOR 30/01/89, August 1989.

Amnesty International. *Torture in the Eighties*. London: AIP, 1984.

Amnesty International Report 1991. London: AI Publications, 1991.

Amnesty International. *Involvement of medical personnel in abuses against detainees and prisoners*. AI Index: ACT 75/08/90, November 1990.

Amnesty International. *Medicine at risk: the doctor as human rights abuser and victim*. London: AI Index: ACT 75/01/89, February 1989.

Amnesty International Medical Commission, Marange V. *Doctors and Torture: Colloboration or Resistance?* London: Bellew, 1991, 166pp. (translated from the French *Médecins tortionnaires, médecins résistants*. Paris: La Decouverte, 1990.)

Amnesty International. *Ethical Codes and Declarations of Relevance to the Health Professions*. London: Amnesty International, 1985.

Apartheid Medicine: Health and Human Rights in South Africa. A report based on a AAAS medical mission of enquiry to South Africa in April 1989. Washington: AAAS, 1990, 131pp.

Beresford D. *Ten Men Dead*. London: Grafton Books, 1987, 432pp.

Bloch S, Reddaway P. *Russia's Political Hospitals: The Abuse of Psychiatry in the Soviet Union*. London: Gollancz, 1977, 510pp.

Bloch S, Reddaway P. *Soviet Psychiatric Abuse: The Shadow over World Psychiatry*. London: Gollancz, 1984, 288pp.

Bloche GM. *Uruguay's Military Physicians: Cogs in a System of State Terror*. Washington: AAAS, 1987, 46pp.

British Medical Association. *Torture Report*. London: BMA, 1986, 34pp.

British Medical Association. *The Handbook of Medical Ethics*, London: BMA, 1984, 111pp.

British Medical Association. *Working Party Report on the Health Care of Remand Prisoners*. London: BMA, 1990, 28pp.

British Medical Association. *Philosophy and Practice of Medicine*. London: BMA, 1988, 137pp.

Burges SH. Doctors and torture: the Police Surgeon. *Journal of Medical Ethics*, 1980, **6**:120-3.

Casscells W, Curran WJ. Doctors, the death penalty and lethal injections; recent developments. *New England Journal of Medicine*, 1982, **307**:1532-3.

Claude P, Stover E, Lopez JP. *Health Professionals and Human Rights in the Philippines*, Washington: American Association for the Advancement of Science, 1987.

Colegio Médico de Chile, *Coloquio Internacional: "Rol de las Asociaciones Médicas en la Defensa de los Derechos Humanos"*. Santiago: CMC, undated [1986].

Colegio Medico de Chile (AG). *Etica Médica: Normas y Documentos [Medical Ethics: Standards and Documents]*. Santiago: Colegio Médico de Chile, 1986, 158pp.

Committee for Health Rights in El Salvador. *Abuses of Medical Neutrality: Report of the Public Health Commission to El Salvador*. Washington, July 1980.

Curran WJ. Casscells W. The ethics of medical participation in capital punishment by intravenous drug injection. *New England Journal of Medicine*, 1980, **302**:226-30.

Doctors, Ethics, and Torture. Proceedings of an International Meeting, Copenhagen, August 1986. *Danish Medical Bulletin*, 1987; **34**:185-216.

van Es A, van Gurp M. *Health Professionals and Human Rights in South Africa*. Report of a mission to the Republic of South Africa on behalf of the Johannes Wier Foundation, 2-15 April 1987. Leiden: Johannes Wier Foundation, 1987, 86pp.

Fireside H. *Soviet Psychoprisons*. New York: Norton, 1979.

Foster D, Davis D, Sandler D. *Detention and Torture in South Africa: psychological, legal and historical studies*. Cape Town: David Philip, 1987, 250pp.

Garfield R, Williams G. *Health and Revolution: The Nicaraguan Experience*. Oxford: Oxfam, 1989, 245pp.

General Medical Council. *Professional Conduct and Discipline: Fitness to Practice*. London: GMC, 1991, 32pp.

Goldstein RH, Breslin P. Technicians of torture: how physicians become agents of state terror. *The Sciences* (New York Academy of Science). March/April 1986, pp. 14-19.

Goldstein R, Gellhorn A. *Human Rights and the Medical Profession in Uruguay Since 1972.* Washington DC: American Association for the Advancement of Science, 1982.

La Grève de la Faim. Paris: Economica, 1984, 173pp.

Gruschow J, Hannibal K (eds). *Health Services for the Treatment of Torture and Trauma Survivors.* Washington: AAAS, 1990, 158pp.

Guatemala: Getting Away With Murder. A report of Americas Watch and Physicians for Human Rights. New York, 1991, 116pp.

Guest I. *Behind the Disappearances: Argentina's Dirty War Against Human Rights and the United Nations.* Philadelphia: University of Pennsylvania Press, 1990, 605pp.

Harding TW. Japan's search for international guidelines on rights of mental patients. *The Lancet*, 1987, i:676-9.

Havard JDJ. Doctors and torture. *British Medical Journal*, 1986, **292**:142-3.

Hood R. *The Death Penalty: a World-wide Perspective.* Oxford: Clarendon Press, 1989, 182pp.

Harding T.W. Prevention of torture and inhuman or degrading treatment: medical implications of a new European convention. *The Lancet*, 1989, i:1191-3.

Human Rights and Mental Patients in Japan. Report of a mission on behalf of the International Commission of Jurists and the International Commission of Health Professionals. Geneva: ICJ, undated [1986], 94pp.

International Committee of the Red Cross. *The Geneva Conventions of August 12 1949.* Geneva: ICRC, 1989, 245pp.

International Committee of the Red Cross. *Protocols Additional to the Geneva Conventions of 12 August 1949.* Geneva: ICRC, 1977, 124pp.

Johannes Wier Foundation. *Health Professionals and Corporal Punishment.* Hague: JWF, 1990.

Kalk WJ, Veriava Y. Hospital management of voluntary total fasting among political prisoners. *Lancet*, 1991; **337**:660-2.

Lifton RJ. *The Nazi Doctors: Medical Killing and the Psychology of Genocide.* London: Papermac, 1986, 561pp.

Manual on the Effective Prevention and Investigation of Extra-legal, Arbitrary and Summary Executions. New York: United Nations, 1991.

Martirena G. *Los médicos y la tortura.* Montevideo: Ediciones de la Banda Oriental, 1988.

Nunca Más. A report by Argentina's National Commission on Disappeared People. London: Faber and Faber, 1986, 463pp.

O'Malley P. *Biting at the Grave: The Irish Hunger Strikes and the Politics of Despair.* Belfast: The Blackstaff Press, 1990, 330pp.

Peters E. *Torture.* Oxford: Basil Blackwell, 1985, 202pp.

Phillips M, Dawson J. *Doctors' Dilemmas: Medical Ethics and Contemporary Science.* Brighton: The Harvester Press, 1985, 230pp.

Proctor R. *Racial Hygiene: Medicine Under the Nazis.* Cambridge: Harvard University Press, 1988.

Radelet ML, Barnard GW. Treating those found incompetent for execution: ethical chaos with only one solution. *Bulletin of the American Academy of Psychiatry and Law*, 1988, **16**:297-308.

Radelet ML, Barnard GW. Ethics and the psychiatric determination of competency to be executed. *Bulletin of the American Academy of Psychiatry and Law*, 1986, **14**:537-553.

Radelet ML, Vandiver M. *Capital Punishment in America: An Annotated Bibliography.* New York: Garland, 1988.

Rasmussen OV. Medical Aspects of Torture. *Danish Medical Bulletin*, 1990; **37** (Supplement 1):1-88.

Rayner M. *Turning a Blind Eye? Medical Accountability and the Prevention of Torture in South Africa.* Washington: AAAS, 1987, 96pp.

Report on Human Rights in El Salvador. Compiled by Americas Watch and the American Civil Liberties Union, January 26th 1982. New York: Vintage House, 1982, 312pp.

Rivas FS. *Traicion a Hipocrates: Médicos en el Aparato Represivo de la Dictadura.* Santiago: CESOC, 1990.

Rodley N. *The Treatment of Prisoners under International Law.* Oxford: OUP, 1987.

Ruthven M. *Torture: The Grand Conspiracy.* London: Weidenfeld and Nicolson, 1978.

Sheleff LS. *Ultimate Penalties: Capital Punishment, Life Imprisonment, Physical Torture.* Columbus: Ohio State University Press, 1987, 492pp.

Silove D. Doctors and the state: lessons from the Biko case. *Social Science and Medicine*, 1990; **30**:417-29.

Sim J. *Medical Power in Prisons: The Prison Medical Service in England, 1774-1989.* Milton Keynes: Open University Press, 1990, 212pp.

Smith R. *Prison Health Care.* London: British Medical Association, 1984, 182 pp.

Stover E. *The Open Secret: Torture and the Medical Profession in Chile.* Washington, AAAS, 1987, 82pp.

Stover E, Nightingale EO (eds). *The Breaking of Bodies and Minds: Torture, Psychiatric Abuse and the Health Professions.* New York: WH Freeman, 1985, 319pp.

Suedfeld P. (ed.) *Psychology and Torture.* New York: Hemisphere, 1990, 207pp.

Thorburn KM. Physicians and the death penalty. *Western Journal of Medicine*, 1987; **146**:638-40.

Timerman J. *Prisoner without a Name, Cell without a Number* (trans. T Talbot). London: Weidenfeld and Nicolson, 1981.

Torture and the Medical Profession. Proceedings of an international symposium, Tromsø, 5-7 June 1990. *Journal of Medical Ethics*, 1991; **17**: Supplement.

Torture in Brazil. A report by the Archdiocese of São Paulo. (Trans. J Wright; Ed. J Dassin). New York: Vintage, 1986, 238pp. Edited English language version of *Brasil: nunca mais.* Petropolis: Editora Vozes, 1985.

United Nations Commission on Human Rights. 43rd Session. Report by the special rapporteur on torture, Professor P Kooijmans (see Chapter 3: Role of Medical Personnel in Torture). UN Doc. E/CN.4/1987/13, 9 January 1987.

Weschler L. *A Miracle, A Universe: Settling Accounts with Torturers.* New York: Pantheon, 1990, 293pp.

Williams P, Wallace D. *Unit 731.* London: Grafton, 1990, 527pp.

Zwi AB. The political abuse of medicine and the challenge of opposing it. *Social Science and Medicine*, 1987; **25**:649-57.

Index

African Charter on Human and
  Peoples' Rights 18
Africa Watch 160
Al-Abub, Dr Aziz 42
AIDS
  compulsory testing 143
  and human rights 143n,177n
Alexandra Clinic 55
Allodi F 29,59
Alvord, Gary, restoring to
  competence for execution 109,
  110
AMA News 113
American Association for the
  Advancement of Science (AAAS)
  xvii,38,156n,174n,191
American College of Physicians 115
American Medical Association (see
  Medical Associations)
American Psychiatric Association
  106
American Psychological Association
  134
Americas Watch 75
Amnesty International xvii,21,23,
  30,31,38,42,44,46,47,51,68,75,95
  138,139,151,154,162,165,180,191
  196
    12-point program for the
    prevention of torture 42,220
amputation, punitive 90-92,94,95
  and religious values 97
Appelbaum PS 105,106n,111n,
  133n
Argentina
  Confederación médica 172
  conviction of doctor 25,59
  death squad 1
Arroyo, Dr Sergio 23
Association of Christians for the
  Abolition of Torture 22,180
Association of Israel-Palestinian
  Physicians for Human Rights 22

asylum seekers 143
Averroes Hospital, Casablanca 127

Balkar Singh, medical examination
  of 54
Bamber, Helen 61
Bassiouni MC 95n
Bawa, Dr Anand Gopal Singh 54
BBC [British Broadcasting
  Corporation]
  television 1,50
  World Service 100,145
Beresford D 125n
Berges, Dr Antonio 25n
Bhutto, Benazir 89
Biko case 139,173,177
Birley, Dr James 71
Bloch S 65,153n
Bloche MG 38,39n,60,132n
Blom-Cooper, Louis 137
Bonnie R 105
Brazil 22,39
  Brasil: Nunca mais 28
British Medical Association
  appeals on human rights cases
    175,207
  ARM decisions 208-210
  policies
    female circumcision 145
    hunger strikes 12
    judicial punishments 11,12
    torture 10,11
  Torture Report xiv,11,40,43,
    176,191,194
  Working Party composition and
    terms of reference, xv
Brown CJ 75n
Bukovsky V 65,75,151n,153
Butler RA 85

Cadogan Committee on corporal
  punishment 85
capital punishment

assessing competence 108-110
bungled executions 114,115
certifying death 116
certifying fitness for execution
 108
development of 98
direct v contributory involvement
 102
evidence in capital trials 104
evidence of Dr James Grigson
 106,107
execution by lethal injection 98,
 99,101,112-114
execution of Rickey Ray Rector
 113,114
hypothetical questions in capital
 trials 106
medical care to condemned
 prisoner 109-111
methods of execution 84
psychiatry, role in 104,105,109,
 110
recommendations 200,201
research into 32
use of organs following 99-102,
 147
Carlisle, Mark 123
Casscells W 98n
Cassidy, Dr Sheila xii
Ceausescu, President 74,112n
Chernin E 146n
Chile 4
 Carabineros, torture by 45
 Central nacional de informaciones
 43
 Colegio Medico de (Chilean
 Medical Association)
 28,34,44,53,57n,61,158
China, People's Republic
 executions and organ use 100
 sterilization 145
Churkin, Dr Alexandr 68
circumcision, female 145,146
Claude RP 52n
Cliff J 165n
Committee for Health Rights in El
 Salvador 156n
Commonwealth Human Rights

Initiative 179,196
Commonwealth of Independent
 States (CIS: see also Union of
 Soviet Socialist Republics) 4,80,
 81
corporal punishment
 BMA policy
 Cadogan Committee 85
 Human Rights Committee on
  13,86,93
 international standards 13,16,86
 in Malaysia 87
 in Pakistan 89
 in Singapore 88
 in South Africa 88
 in Sudan 90
 in the UK 84,85
 recommendations 201,202
Council of Europe 182
Council of International
 Organizations of Medical Sciences
 14
Cowgill G 29,59
Cuba, reports of psychiatric abuse
 74,75
Curran WJ 98n, 112n
Czechoslovakia 4,66

Davis, Dr Paul 55
Dawson, Dr John xiii,xiv,43n,
 144n,176,185n
death penalty (see capital
 punishment)
Declaration of Geneva 15
Declaration of Hawaii 14
Declaration of Kuwait 15
Declaration of Madrid 17
Declaration of Tokyo xi,11-
 13,33,40,45,94,121,130,166,
 170,172,210
Deva, Prof P 71
Devlin, Lord 9
"doubling" 37
Duhamel O 121n

East Timor, torture xii
Eisenberg C 156n
El Salvador, torture in 46

van Es A 55n
Esperson O 181n
European Commission of Human
    Rights 135
European Committee for the
    Prevention of Torture 79,188,195
European Convention for the
    Prevention of Torture, 17,86
European Convention for the
    Protection of Human Rights 19
European Court of Human Rights
    185n,186
European Principles of Medical
    Ethics 14
European Prison Rules 17
executions (see capital punishment)
experimentation on prisoners 146

Fadul, Dr Ali, death under torture
    6,160,175
Fisher, Dr Fleur 176
flogging, see corporal punishment
forcible feeding 120,123-127
forcible medical examination 141,
    142
Freeman v Home Office 137
Fuenzalida, Dr Luis Losada, issuing
    of false medical certificate 57

Gardiner, Lord 45
Garfield R 164n
General Medical Council (GMC) 10
Geneva Conventions of 1949 15,16
    Protocols to 15,16
di Georgi S 182n
German Democratic Republic 7,26,
    76
Greece, see Leros
Gibson J 36
Gillon R   15n
Gluzman, Dr Semyon 5,30,65,66,
    73,153-155
Goldstein R 171n
GRAPO, hunger strikes 125-127
Greece, torture trials 25
Grigorenko, Gen. Piotr 4,73,152,
    153
Grigson, Dr James 106

Grivnina I 153
Grove R 77n
Gruschow J 205n
Guest I 2n
Gunn J 137n
van Gurp M 55n

Hamilton G 169n
Handbook of Medical Ethics 12
Hannibal K 205n
Haritos-Fatouros M 36
Havard, Dr John 176
Health Advisory Service 80,190
health workers
    attacks on, in:
        Chile 157,158
        China 158
        El Salvador 155
        Mozambique 165
        Nicaragua 164
        Sudan 160
        Syria 153
        Turkey 161
        USSR 151-3
        Vietnam 159
        Yugoslavia 163
    protection of 165-7,203
Helsinki Watch 30
Hidalgo, Ariel, experience in
    Havana Psychiatric Hospital 75,76
Hong Kong, use of organs from
    executed prisoners 100
Hopkins H 83n,93n
Howard League for Penal Reform
    142n
Hu H 140n
Human Rights Committee of UN
    13,86,93
Hungary 4,66
hunger strikes
    BMA policy 12
    deaths as a result of 124-127
    evolution of policy in UK 122-4
    in Morocco 127,128
    in N. Ireland 120
    in Spain 125-127
    in South Africa 128,129
    recommendations 197

treatment of hunger-strikers 120
Hussain, Dr Mohamed 6,160,175

Illinois State Medical Society 113
India
    pressure to falsify evidence 55
    proposal for lethal injection 114
    Punjab, alleged torture 53
International Association on the
    Political Abuse of Psychiatry
    30,31n,66n
International Commission of
    Health Professionals 78,180
International Commission of Jurists
    78,180
International Commission on
    Medical Neutrality 157
International Committee of the
    Red Cross (ICRC) 15n,150,180,
    196
International Council of Nurses
    14,179
International Covenant on Civil and
    Political Rights (ICCPR) 18
International Federation of Human
    Rights 22
International Helsinki Federation for
    Human Rights xiin
International Organization against
    Torture 22
International Tribunal for the
    Investigation of Torture 181
intimate body searches 141,142
Iran, and death penalty 84n
Iraq, ex-sanguination of prisoners
    103n
Isle of Man, corporal punishment 86
Israel
    Association of Israel-Palestinian
        Physicians for Human Rights
        58n
    pregnant prisoner bound to bed 58

Japan,
    and capital punishment 31
    psychiatric practice 77,78
    war crimes 25,146n
Jenkins, Roy 123

Johannes Wier Foundation,
    Netherlands xvii,48n,73n,87n,
    95n,147n,180

Kalk WJ 128
Kashmir xi,21
Kooijmans, Prof. Peter 2n,5,62,97
Koryagin, Dr Anatoly 153,166
Kosovo, beatings of prisoners 48,
    49
Kuwait
    attacks on health workers 162
    torture of Palestinians 50

Leros, psychiatric institution,
    Greece 77
Lexington High Security Unit, USA
    142
Lifton RJ 35,37
Lin Yeong-fan, Dr 101
Lök V 28n
Lopez JP 52n
Lore C 182n

Malaysia
    corporal punishment 87
Malzfeldt, Dr Claudia 8n,27
Marange V 184n
Martirena, Dr Gregorio 28n,60n,
    172n
Mauritania
    amputations 94
    AMPHOM 94
    Red Crescent 51
    torture in 51
McDougall, Mrs Barbara 133
Médecins du Monde 180
Médecins sans Frontières 180
Medical Associations
    America, United States (AMA)
        98,112,116
    Argentina 172
    Brazil 169
    Britain (see BMA)
    Canada 177
    Chile 34,44,53,57n,61,158,166,
        169,170,171n
    Commonwealth 179,196

Denmark 181,199
South Africa 129n,173,174
Sweden 132
Syria 154,155
Turkey 173
Uruguay 171,181,199
medical care
  withholding from prisoners 138-
  140,161
medical ethics
  inadequate understanding 40
  standards 10-16
  recommendations 198,199
Medical Foundation for the Care of
  Victims of Torture 7,52,61, 180
Medvedev Z 151n
Mehdi, Dr Mahboob 89,97
Mental Health Act Commission 190
Merritt J 77n
Middle East Watch 162
Mielke F 25n,146n
Milgram S x,35n
Mitscherlich A 25n,146n
Montevideo group 181
Morocco, hunger strikes in 127
Mozambique, attacks on health
  personnel 165
Mustafa, Dr Kamil Zaki 91

Nadvi S, 93n
National Commission of Medical
  Ethics, Uruguay 28,61
Nazi crimes 146
Netherlands
  position on corporal punishment
  96,202
  'doctors of confidence' 131
Nightingale EO 152n,184n
Nguyen Dan Que, Dr,
  imprisonment of 159
Nicaragua, attacks on health
  personnel 164
Nordic medical associations,
  declaration on death penalty 116
Northern Ireland
  1981 hunger strikes 120,121,
  124,125
Nunca Más 28

Official Secrets Act 185
Olivares, Dr Ramiro, imprisonment
  of 56,158
Olubodun JOB 140n
O'Malley P 125n,131n
Organization of African Unity
  (OAU) 18
Orr, Dr Wendy 174

Pakistan
  corporal punishment 89
  Pakistan Medical Assn. 95n
  Qisas and Diyat Ordinance 89,90
  Voice Against Torture 89,95n
Parker Committee 40
Peters E 83n
Petersen HD 47,60
Phillips M 43n,144n,185n
*Philosophy and Practice of Medical
  Ethics* 10,11
Physicians for Human Rights
  PHR Denmark 180
  PHR USA xvii,48n,157,159,162,
  163,165,180
  PHR UK xvii,21,180
Plyusch L 151n
Pogliano C 182n
Principles of Medical Ethics 13,
  14,45,94,177
Proctor R 146n
Punjab, torture in 53
psychiatry
  abuse of 30,65,66
  and the death penalty
  104,105,109,110
  US delegation to USSR 69,70
  WPA delegation to USSR 71,192

Raat A-M 127n
Radelet, Prof. Michael 108,109n,
  110n
Rasmussen, OV 29,60,132n
Rayner M 139n,174n
Rector, Rickey Ray, execution of
  113,114
Red Crescent, Mauritania 51
Red Cross (see International
  Commission of the Red Cross)

Reddaway P 65,66n,67,69n,71n,
153n
Reeve PA 140n
Reich W 152n
Renamo 42,165
Reyes H 181n
Rich V 73n
Rivas F 171n
Rodley N 14n,16n,20n,86n,94
Romania 4,66
Roth, Prof. Loren 71
Royal College of Psychiatrists 30,
72n

Santibañez, Federico Alvarez, death
under torture 57
schizophrenia, in the USSR 70
Seelman, Dr Gunter 171n
Sendero Luminoso 42
Serbia, abuses against ethnic
Albanians xii,48,49,163
Serbsky Institute 152
shari'a 87,90,95
Sharma, Dr RK 55
Sheleff LS 99
Shibata, Dr Harry 39,169
Sieghart P 143n
Silove D 174n
Shu-Hsu Chu, Prof. 101
Sim J 138n
Singapore, and corporal punishment
88
Siu-Keung Lam 100n
Smith R 56n,119n,137n
South Africa
Medical Association of South
Africa 129n,173-175
Medical and Dental Council 174
National Medical and Dental
Association 129n,175
Sri Lanka, human rights violations,
xi
Stasi 8,26
Staub E 36,37
sterilization, forcible 144,145
Stover E 35n,38n,152n,170n,171n,
184n
strip searching

in N Ireland 142
in USA 142
Sudan
death of Dr Ali Fadul 6,160,175
death sentence on doctor 6,160,
175
punitive amputations 90-92
SWAPO [South West Africa
People's Organization] 42
Swedish Medical Association 132
Syria, 7
Bar Association, 7
detained physicians, 7
Ordre des médecins syriens
(medical association) 154,155,
173

Taiwan
executions and organ transplants
100,101,115
National Taiwan Hospital 101
Tantam D 65n
Ternovsky, Dr Leonard 153
Timerman, Jacobo 1,24
torture
BMA report xiv,11,40,43,176,
191,194
definition of medical involvement
34
issuing false certificates after 53,
57,58
medical examination before 42-45
medical presence during 45-49
"Tucker telephone" 33
Tuffs, Annette 26n
Tumim, Judge Stephen 188
Turkey
arrest of TMA members 173
chaining of prisoners to beds 58
conflict with PKK 51
torture of doctors 161,162
torture and medical neglect 46,47
Tyrer case, Isle of Man 86

Union of Soviet Socialist Republics
(USSR: see also Commonwealth
of Independent States)
psychiatric abuse 31,65-73

All-Union Society of Psychiatrists
and Narcologists 67,71,72,172
prosecution of opponents 151-153
United Kingdom
corporal punishment 84,85
European Committee for the
Prevention of Torture, report
188
Health Advisory Service 80
HM Chief Inspector of Prisons
xi,188
hunger strikes 120,122-124
Mental Health Act Commission
79
psychiatry 79,80
United Nations
Body of Principles 16,42
Convention against Torture 16
Declaration on the Protection of
all Persons from being
subjected to torture 17
Human Rights Commission xi,19
Human Rights Committee 13,86,
93
International Covenant on Civil
and Political Rights 18,86,93
Principles of Medical Ethics
13,14,45,94,177
Principles for the Protection of
Persons with Mental Illness
17,81,82,138,149
Special Rapporteur on Torture
2,5,54,62,97,191
Standard Minimum Rules for the
Treatment of Prisoners 17,
86,94
Uruguay 7,61
Federación Médica del Interior
171
National Commission of Medical
Ethics 34,61
Sindicato Médico 171

van Voren, R 71n
Venezuela 47
Dirección de Inteligencia Militar
48
Veriava Y 128

Vesti P 29
Vicaria de la Solidaridad 56,158
Vietnam, imprisonment of doctor
159
Vines A 165n
virginity testing 144
Voice Against Torture 85,95n
Voloshanovich, Dr Alexander 153

Wakley, Dr Thomas, on corporal
punishment 93
Wallace D 146n
Washington v. Harper 133
Weschler L 60n,132n
West LJ 105n
Wheeler, Charles 50
whipping (see corporal punishment)
Whitehead, Dr Tony 138n
Williams G 164n
Williams P 146n
Wilson, Dr Tim 55
Wiseberg L 165n
World Health Organization 14,176
World Medical Association 112,
122,131,141,155,166,177,187,
196
Declarations 11,12,13,33,45,94,
121,130,166,170,172,193
and hunger strikes 121,122
Secretary-General 99
World Psychiatric Association
14,178,179,192
visit to USSR 71,72
Wynen, Dr André 166n,178

Yugoslavia
abuses in Kosovo 165
beatings of Albanians 48,49
arrest of doctor, Croatia 166
psychiatric abuse 4,66

Zimbardo PG 36n

Zed Books Ltd

is a publisher whose international and Third World lists span:

- **Women's Studies**
- **Development**
- **Environment**
- **Current Affairs**
- **International Relations**
- **Children's Studies**
- **Labour Studies**
- **Cultural Studies**
- **Human Rights**
- **Indigenous Peoples**
- **Health**

We also specialize in Area Studies where we have extensive lists in African Studies, Asian Studies, Caribbean and Latin American Studies, Middle East Studies, and Pacific Studies.

For further information about books available from Zed Books, please write to: Catalogue Enquiries, Zed Books Ltd, 57 Caledonian Road, London N1 9BU. Our books are available from distributors in many countries (for full details, see our catalogues), including:

In the USA
Humanities Press International, Inc., 165 First Avenue,
Atlantic Highlands, New Jersey 07716.
Tel: (908) 872 1441;
Fax: (908) 872 0717.

In Canada
Garamond Press, Suite 408, 77 Mowat Avenue, Toronto,
Ontario M6K 3E3.
Tel: (416) 516 2709.

In Australia
Peribo Pty Ltd, 26 Tepko Road, Terrey Hills, NSW 2084.

In Southern Africa
David Philip Publisher (Pty) Ltd, PO Box 408, Claremont 7735,
South Africa.